W9-APC-993

Policies and Procedures

for Infusion Nursing of the Older Adult

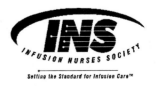

INFUSION NURSES SOCIETY

Setting the Standard for Infusion Care™

Many older adults require infusion therapy for medical management of a variety of acute or chronic diseases or conditions. When caring for the older adult, it is important to understand physiologic changes that occur as a result of aging processes and the possible effects those changes may have on infusion-related outcomes. Such knowledge will enable the nurse to adapt infusion techniques and interventions to accommodate special infusion care needs of the older adult.

The Infusion Nurses Society (INS) recognizes that the majority of patients are receiving therapies in multiple care settings, such as acute care, long-term care and homecare. Due to their specialized care requirements and needs, it is important that the nurse become more informed about the older adult population.

INS has developed *Policies and Procedures for Infusion Nursing of the Older Adult* as a result of a grant award from the Nurse Competence in Aging initiative funded by the Atlantic Philanthropies, and supported by American Nurses Association, American Nurses Credentialing Center and the John A. Hartford Foundation's Institute for Geriatric Nursing.

Policies and Procedures for Infusion Nursing of the Older Adult serves as a clinical care guide and provides the nurse with information necessary to provide quality infusion care specific to the older adult population.

- **Assessment** of the older adult is presented as an introduction and supplies information that may affect infusion therapy modalities when caring for the older adult population.
- **Considerations** for the older adult, which are noted at the beginning of each policy, are intended to enhance nursing knowledge that is specific to the older adult receiving infusion therapy administration.
- **Policies** describe courses and purposes of indicated actions while **Procedures** details particular steps to be undertaken to achieve intended outcomes.

Note:
The healthcare organization that uses this manual should be aware that annual review of organizational polices and procedures should continue to occur in accordance and compliance with regulatory and nonregulatory agencies.

These policies and procedures are voluntary, advisory guidelines. An independent review and assessment should be conducted to determine applicability and appropriateness to the clinical setting. Infusion therapies present risks, and it is the responsibility of the healthcare organization to manage these risks, including skills and competency validation of personnel.

Copyright ©2004 by the Infusion Nurses Society. All rights reserved. No part of this manual may be reproduced without written permission from the Infusion Nurses Society, 220 Norwood Park South, Norwood, MA 02062.

Table of Contents

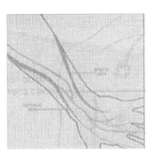

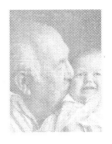

1.

Assessment of the Older Adult Receiving Infusion Therapy

The Older Adult

Older adults may require infusion therapy for a variety of conditions or diagnostic indications. An assessment, includes a system-by-system examination: a review of medical, medication, and infusion therapy history; confirmation of ability to perform activities of daily living (ADLs); and psychological and safety assessments. Contact information, family and community resources, and advance directives should also be included in the assessment.

The following is a summary of considerations that may affect infusion device selection, vascular access site care and management strategies, and anticipated outcomes.

Physiological Changes and Infusion Considerations

INTEGUMENTARY SYSTEM

Many changes occur in the integumentary system of older adults that can have a significant impact on the provision of infusion therapy services. As the individual ages, there is a decrease in the body's water content. This, in addition to a loss of subcutaneous fat, makes the skin dry and loose. The number of sweat cells decreases and diminish in efficiency as less sebum is produced. This results in a decreased ability to perspire, further enhancing skin dryness. Skin will appear looser, as the number of papillae (the cells that hold the three layers of the skin tightly together) decreases.

Sensory changes that can accompany aging may cause a decrease in the thirst reflex mechanism, and lead to dehydration. Hydration imbalances may make skin turgor evaluation a poor assessment tool. Hydration as a form of "pretreatment" may be necessary before infusion therapy can be initiated.

The number of sensory nerve endings decrease with age as does the older adult's ability to perceive pain. This increases the risk that an individual's reaction to skin damage will be delayed or will go unnoticed. Should a medication or solution infiltrate into the underlying tissues, it may not be immediately recognized. This can lead to a delay in treating the infiltration, increasing potential damage to the tissues.

The epidermis becomes thin and inelastic with age. Collagen fibers decrease in number and function, contributing to the skin's loss of flexibility and elasticity. The epidermis is also rendered more fragile and heals more slowly as skin cell turnover rate decreases. Looser skin and a loss of subcutaneous tissue make the veins less stable, and a thinner surface makes the skin more fragile, increasing risk of skin tears. This thinning outer skin layer is a much less effective barrier against the introduction of microorganisms.

Capillaries also decrease in number giving the skin a translucent, almost transparent appearance. The integrity of the capillary wall is altered as cells lose water content, become less elastic and more rigid. This, in turn, makes them fragile, increasing the risk of bruising and vein rupture during venipuncture.

Metabolic imbalances serve as comorbidities and may impact infusion therapy treatment. Some metabolic imbalances may be due to the aging process itself, but others may be a result of kidney, liver, or endocrine conditions such as diabetes mellitus, cholelithiasis, or hyperthyroidism. Decrease in water content, when observed as physical changes, may be due to changes in function of the pituitary and thyroid glands. An increase in pruritis, or dry, itchy skin may occur. Pruritis may also occur as an adverse medication reaction.

The vascular access device (VAD) insertion technique and site dressing materials should accommodate the older adult's more fragile skin and vascular access status. To minimize bruising, extreme care should be taken when applying a tourniquet. The patient's infusion history should address phlebitis or infiltration occurrences associated with previous infusions, and document any allergic reactions to adhesives, adhesive removers, and skin disinfecting solutions.

The nurse should select an area with adequate tissue to provide catheter stabilization. The impact of vein conservation on future vascular access should be considered. Catheter threading may be difficult if the vein lumen has narrowed due to venous wall thickening or deposits of calcium or plaque. Diminished blood return leads to slower venous distention. This may affect flashback, so care should be taken when advancing the catheter.

IMMUNE SYSTEM

The aging immune system becomes hyporesponsive to foreign antigens but hyperresponsive to self. This leads to a decrease in circulating lymphocytes, a decreased production of inter-leukin-2, fewer cytokine receptors, and an increased production of antigens. Immunologic cellular function declines, increasing the risk of developing cancers and autoimmune disorders.

A system less responsive to pathogenic microorganisms decreases the older adult's resistance to infection, placing him or her at increased risk for nosocomial infections. Adherence to correct hand hygiene practices, attention to aseptic technique, and proper site preparation become especially important infusion nursing practices as the patient's susceptibility to infection rises.

Common signs of infection may be altered in the older adult. Cell turnover rate decreases, leading to an increase in the length of time for general healing. Healing not only takes longer, but may not be as complete. For example, fever may be delayed or absent a few days after the onset of an infection. Infection may present in the form of disorientation, delirium (acute change in mental status), decreased appetite, decreased ability to conduct ADLs, loss of bladder control, or lethargy.

MUSCULOSKELETAL SYSTEM

The musculoskeletal system is affected both structurally and functionally with aging. Cartilage composition changes and lean muscle mass decreases. This decrease can be compounded if accompanied by a lowered protein intake stemming from a decrease in appetite. Wear and tear on articulating surfaces increases the risk of developing osteoarthritis. Cellular changes in muscle mass, ligaments, tendons, and cartilage result in a loss of elasticity, increasing overall body stiffness. This can further lead to decreased mobility, strength, and endurance resulting in increased risk of falls and fractures.

Immobility or decreased mobility places the older adult at greater risk for development of multiple conditions including, but not limited to, joint and muscle stiffness and pain, pneumonia, pressure ulcers, decreased appetite resulting in undernutrition, decreased fluid intake that causes dehydration, and potential deep vein thrombosis with risk of pulmonary embolism.

Consideration of the older adult's decreased mobility should be a part of the infusion therapy plan of care. This includes attention to ambulation with an electronic infusion device (EID), length of tubing selected, site selection on the nondominant arm, and the use of armboards. In the immobile patient, proper positioning is especially important. Attention must be paid to prevent impeding circulation or venous stasis that could contribute to the development of deep vein thrombosis or pulmonary embolism.

An assessment of the patient's manual dexterity is especially important when evaluating the older adult infusion patient for appropriateness of home-based infusion therapy. Impaired joint mobility affects the ability to handle a syringe, draw up a medication or flush solution, or connect a syringe to an administration port or cap.

DIGESTIVE SYSTEM

Medical causes of poor nutrition such as swallowing difficulties, hand tremors, muscle weakness or paralysis, or cognitive impairment should be assessed. Nutritional assessments should include the social aspects of eating, including the ability to shop for and prepare food, or self-feed.

Age-related gastrointestinal changes, poor dentition, and tooth loss place the older adult at increased risk for malnutrition which slows wound healing. Stomach motility is decreased and emptying of the stomach is delayed resulting in a feeling of fullness before the patient has had adequate nutrient intake. Early satiety can result in inadequate fluid intake, causing fluid and electrolyte imbalance. Medications with diuretic functions can further lower potassium levels, increasing the need to monitor potassium intake and serum levels. Immobility resulting from joint and muscle pain, stiffness, and chronic medical conditions increases the older adult's need for protein.

Diminished hepatocellular functioning leads to a decrease in liver mass and liver function. Decreased blood flow to the liver alters the rate of drug metabolism, placing the older adult at risk for elevated drug levels in the blood, potential drug toxicities, and subsequent adverse effects. When assessing the older adult patient for infusion therapy, the infusion nurse should consider the possibility of impaired drug metabolism.

RESPIRATORY SYSTEM

Age-related lung changes can lead to impaired oxygen exchange. Changes in these processes will often contribute to confusion and restlessness. Confusion in an older adult should raise concerns about safety in the initiation and continuation of infusion therapies, strategies, and practices.

Joint and muscle stiffness discussed above in "Musculoskeletal System" affects the respiratory system by causing chest wall stiffness, fragility, and loss of lung elasticity. Compromised breathing can affect patient mobility and lead to immobility-related complications. Respiratory infections may persist due to deceased muscle strength of the diaphragm and intercostals muscles and can also contribute to catheter-related infections.

CARDIOVASCULAR SYSTEM

Aging causes the cardiovascular system to become slower in responding to shifts in fluid balance, including the elimination of excess fluid. Nurses caring for older patients with compromised cardiovascular functioning should pay particular attention to the properties of the infusion solution and to the rate of administration to avoid fluid volume deficits.

Sclerosing of cardiac and cerebral vascular networks also suggests that these processes are prevalent in the peripheral vascular network. Peripheral networks are preferred locations for short-term VADs, but catheter penetration through vessel walls may be more difficult. Nurses should adapt to a diminished "bounce" on palpation of distended vessels, and expect slower venous filling.

NEUROLOGICAL SYSTEM

Nurses may encounter older adults coping with dementia, Parkinson's disease, strokes, peripheral neuropathies, and neuropathic pain management. An assessment of dementia, if evident, should differentiate it from those conditions that result from reversible causes such as adverse drug effects, depression, pernicious anemia, and autoimmune and endocrine disorders.

Changes in the functioning of neuroreceptors and overall brain activity may lead to changes in short-term memory. The loss of neurons and slowed neurotransmission results in diminished sensory functioning, slowed reflexes, and increased visual and hearing deficits.

Hearing deficits include difficulty discriminating sounds, especially high-frequency sounds, which can increase the risk of falls or accidents. Older adults with hearing deficits may benefit from an electronic infusion device (EID) with special visual alarms to supplement auditory alarms. Choice of patient education materials should meet the needs of the visually- or hearing-impaired patient. New learning will require more time and should be considered when planning the patient's infusion-specific education.

Neurological deficits can result in loss of cognitive functioning. Older adults with memory deficits may understand the reason for infusion therapy and provide informed consent and yet later forget why they have the device. Patients with delirium may not be able to follow instructions or directions. This may lead the patient to attempt to remove the VAD. If the ability to obtain informed consent is in question, a cognitive assessment becomes critical.

GENITOURINARY SYSTEM

A decrease in body water content impairs fluid and electrolyte balance. Diminished cardiac functioning slows the body's response to increases in fluid and affects fluid excretion. These changes increase the risk for fluid volume deficits that can occur with parenteral fluid administration. Thus, it is important for the nurse to pay special attention to medication and infusate administration rates.

With aging, creatinine clearance slows. Diminished renal functioning slows excretion of medication, increasing the risk of toxic drug build-up in the body. A thorough knowledge of medications excreted via the kidneys allows the nurse to properly assess the patient for potential complications related to drug toxicity.

Bladder capacity and sensation decrease, and residual volumes increase the risk of urinary incontinence. Incontinence and decreased physical mobility increase the risk of urinary tract infections (UTIs). Remote infections such as UTIs have been determined as a potential source for vascular catheter-related infections.

PSYCHOLOGICAL ASSESSMENT

A complete patient assessment will include evaluation of psychological and cognitive functioning, as well as evaluation for depression. Thorough assessment will determine if the older adult is compromised in his or her ability to understand the requirements of infusion therapy, provide informed consent, and comply with prescribed therapy. The need for direct patient supervision during infusion therapy should also be considered. The psychological impact from any hearing or visual deficits, or impaired capacity to independently provide self-care should also be addressed. An older adult may become disoriented and confused when transported from his or her residence to a new care facility. Establishing a baseline functioning level is important in determining the patient's true disorientation or confusion.

ENVIRONMENTAL ASSESSMENT

Nurses will care for older adults in a variety of settings: home, hospital, outpatient, or long-term care facility. A safety evaluation should be part of the environmental assessment. Sensory and motor deficits or impaired functioning of body systems can result in an inability to maintain a safe care setting.

To safely receive home infusion services, a patient must be able to provide a clean area for storage of supplies, including solutions or medications that must be kept refrigerated. Continuous infusion administration should not interfere with the older adult's ability to freely ambulate, negotiate stairs, or provide self-care.

An assessment of the home environment should also indicate the role that the spouse or significant other, family, friends, and community will play in providing care and support for the older patient.

SUMMARY

Overall assessment of the older adult is an essential first step in providing safe and effective infusion care. Physiological changes brought on by the aging process need not prevent quality infusion care as long as the nurse is aware of potential problems, and assesses the patient thoroughly prior to initiation of therapy.

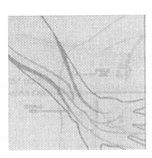

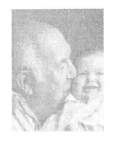

2.

Patient Care

Patient Assessment

> ### CONSIDERATIONS FOR THE OLDER ADULT
>
> Older adults may present with infusion-related issues that affect care planning and intended outcomes. The nurse should ascertain through a careful interview such information as previous infusion history, handedness, ambulation mode, current medical condition and healthcare perceptions of the patient. If necessary, family members or other care providers will also be able to contribute information to guide the assessment process. During the process of assessment, cognitive abilities or disabilities can also be determined and incorporated in the infusion plan of care.

POLICY

Patient assessment is an ongoing process of observation requiring evaluation and judgement by the nurse in order to achieve desired outcomes. Patient assessment shall be documented in the patient's permanent medical record and verbally reported to the physician or legally authorized prescriber, and to other members of the healthcare team as appropriate.

PROCEDURE

1. Verify patient's identity.
2. Obtain and review physician's or legally authorized prescriber's order for infusion therapy.
3. Inform patient of the process.
4. Place patient in a comfortable reclining position, as tolerated, during assessment.
5. Review patient's past and present medical history including:
   - Age
   - Diagnosis
   - Current status
   - Adverse effects or events
   - Allergies
   - Transfusion history
   - Medications
   - Healthcare proxy and advanced directives
6. Review laboratory data including:
   - Electrolytes, serum proteins, nutritional deficiencies, and other assays
   - Renal function tests
   - Radiologic examinations
7. Perform assessments of the following:
   - Height, weight, and body surface area
   - Systems assessment including:
     - Fluid balance and hydration considerations
     - Nutritional status
     - Pain threshold
     - Signs and symptoms of deficiency states
     - Sleep patterns

- Ambulatory aids
- Vital signs
- Vascular system integrity

8. Document assessment on appropriate form in patient's permanent medical record.

9. Perform reassessment at established intervals, and when there is a change in the patient's status, needs, or treatment plan.

Physician's Order

> ## CONSIDERATIONS FOR THE OLDER ADULT
>
> Infusion therapy is initiated and discontinued upon a physician's order or upon the order of a legally authorized prescriber. Safety measures, such as use of electronic infusion devices should be considered when initiating the physician's order for infusion therapy. The older adult will often experience cardiovascular, renal, or hepatic changes associated with aging, and is at increased risk for fluid overload and altered drug metabolism or excretion leading to drug toxicity. Age-related physiological changes necessitate frequent patient monitoring for cognitive or physical side effects of prescribed parenteral medications and infusates. Older adults are also at increased risk for drug-disease, drug-drug, or drug-nutrient interactions, and adverse reactions and events.

POLICY

The nurse must be knowledgeable about state regulations and facility-specific policies and procedures regarding physician's orders pertaining to infusion therapy. In reviewing the physician's orders, the nurse must make sure that none of the orders is in conflict with documented patient advance directives.

The nurse shall not accept an order to Keep Vein Open (KVO) as it is considered incomplete and nonspecific, thereby increasing the risk of infusion-related complications such as fluid overload.

PROCEDURE

1. Written Orders

Prior to the initiation of infusion therapy, a written physician's or legally authorized prescriber's order shall be obtained. If the physician's order is not clear, legible, or complete, the nurse must contact the prescriber for clarification. This order shall contain the following information:

- Parenteral solution or medication to be administered
- Dose
- Volume to be infused
- Rate of administration
- Frequency of administration
- Route of administration
- Anticipated duration of therapy

Verbal Orders

When a physician or legally authorized prescriber gives a verbal order, it shall be written and signed by the physician or legally authorized prescriber in the appropriate amount of time.

Discontinuing Therapy

To discontinue infusion therapy, a written order must be signed by a physician or legally authorized prescriber.

In the Hospital Setting

Orders taken from a physician or legally authorized prescriber by a registered nurse (RN) shall be written by the RN and signed by the physician or legally authorized prescriber within 24 hours.

In the Alternative Care Setting

Verbal orders taken in the alternative care setting must be sent to the physician or legally authorized prescriber for signature. A written and signed order must be in the patient's medical record within 30 days.

Informed Consent

CONSIDERATIONS FOR THE OLDER ADULT

Before informed consent can be obtained, it is necessary to assess the older adult's mental status. Mental status can be impaired for many reasons. If impaired memory or confusion is due to a reversible condition, it is important to address the underlying condition. If pain is affecting the older adult's ability to think clearly, appropriate management strategies must be in place prior to obtaining informed consent.

The nurse should assess any sensory deficits, such as vision or hearing, provide written consent forms that are printed in an easy-to-read font, and adapt spoken information for any hearing deficits. The use of unfamiliar language should be avoided, and written material should be provided at the patient's reading level. Pausing periodically allows the patient time to process the information given and can enhance comprehension. The nurse may have to adapt the signed consent process if the older adult has developed upper extremity problems, such as fine tremors, poor eye-hand coordination or range-of-motion limitations.

The nurse must be knowledgeable about advance directives and existing healthcare proxies.

POLICY

The patient's informed consent shall be obtained before initiating infusion therapy. In the event that a patient is deemed incompetent or unable to give consent, the consent of a legally authorized representative shall be obtained. It is the responsibility of the organization to determine which infusion therapies require informed consent.

PROCEDURE

1. Verify patient's identity.
2. Obtain and review physician's or legally authorized prescriber's order for infusion therapy.
3. Obtain appropriate informed consent form.
4. Provide patient with information regarding the ordered therapy in a language and at an education level understood by the patient.
5. Allow opportunity for dialogue between the patient or representative and nurse regarding the information provided.
6. Obtain patient's or legally authorized representative's signature on informed consent form.
7. Place signed and dated informed consent form in the patient's permanent medical record.

Unusual Occurrence Reporting

CONSIDERATIONS FOR THE OLDER ADULT

The older adult presents special concerns in terms of patient safety. Documentation of the older adult's physical, physiological, and cognitive deficits or limitations facilitates the evaluation of potential injury and its implications for the patient's health.

Additional considerations for Unusual Occurrence Reporting include, but are not limited to, adverse or untoward reactions to parenteral medications or infusates, injury resulting from parenteral medication- and infusion-related errors and injury resulting from infusion devices or equipment due to catheter insertion, break in aseptic technique, or equipment defect or malfunction.

POLICY

An Unusual Occurrence Report shall be used to document an unusual and unanticipated occurrence or variance resulting in actual or potential injury or harm. The organization shall determine the proper documentation form and the mechanism to report incidents. Unusual Occurrence Reports shall require appropriate follow-up and documentation of any corrective action taken. Confidentiality of information contained within the Unusual Occurrence Report shall be maintained in a manner determined by the organization.

PROCEDURE

Preparing an Unusual Occurrence Report

When preparing an Unusual Occurrence Report, the nurse must document the objective account of the event including:

1. Type of occurrence or variance
2. Assessment of patient's condition before and after the occurrence or variance
3. Follow-up and corrective actions taken

After Documenting an Unusual Occurrence

1. Notify patient's physician and other members of the healthcare team as appropriate.
2. Maintain confidentiality of information; do not put the completed Unusual Occurrence Report, or reference to report, in patient's medical record.
3. Analyze data for trends as determined by the organization or regulatory or accrediting agency.

Patient Education

CONSIDERATIONS FOR THE OLDER ADULT

Patient education not only provides information to enable the older adult to be more knowledgeable about his or her condition, but it facilitates educated participation in self-care practices. Slowed mental functioning does not necessarily mean that comprehension is impaired, but it does require a slower pace of teaching. Depression can also slow mental processing, and must be assessed if suspected.

Assessing the older adult's and caregiver's emotional, cognitive and physical capacities to provide and participate in infusion therapy is an important first step. Patient education may involve not only the older adult but a spouse, grown children or other family members, friends, or other caregivers.

Aging anatomy and physiology results in many changes that can adversely impact the older adult's ability to communicate, participate in, and benefit from education sessions.

The goals and objectives for each teaching session should be clear to both the nurse and the learner. The older adult may have different teaching needs for infusion therapy than the caregiver.

- Determine the older adult's or caregiver's preexisting knowledge of the information to be conveyed.
- Speak clearly and distinctly, and avoid unfamiliar terminology. Speak slowly and in a low-toned voice if the older adult has a hearing impairment. Avoid shouting, which can distort sound. Facing the older adult prevents him or her from having to turn sideways to make eye contact, which prevents potential neck strain and also helps to compensate for losses in peripheral vision.
- Consider the use of videotaped teaching materials as a reinforcement of education.
- If the older adult uses a hearing aid, make sure it is in place, with fully functioning batteries.
- Include the patient in conversation, even when the focus of the session is on teaching a caregiver.
- Select written materials that are in an easy-to-read font. Large print medication labels should be considered. Use of all capital letters or italics can be more difficult to read. A magnifying glass can improve legibility, unless manual dexterity is compromised. Overhead lighting can minimize glare.
- Select teaching materials that are at the appropriate reading level of the older adult.
- When designing materials for patient education, prepare printed material with double-spaced lines, and wide, print-free margins. Consider the use of illustrated charts and tables. Materials printed on matte—not glossy paper—are easier to read.
- Present information in a logical step-by-step format, in the same sequence as will be necessary to complete the task.
- Try to individualize the teaching materials to the specific needs of the older adult whenever possible.

Continued

- Demonstrate procedures in addition to describing them. Reinforce or review information frequently and reassess whether teaching has been effective. Pausing allows time to process the information, and decreases the risk of confusing one concept with another.
- Keep education sessions short.
- Request return demonstrations to allow the older adult the opportunity to work through the procedure with the nurse present. Individuals retain more content from instruction with return demonstration than from just reading or listening to information.
- As difficulties arise, allow the older adult the opportunity to problem-solve and find creative solutions.
- Manual dexterity may be compromised and may make it more difficult to manipulate small objects such as injection caps.
- Consider the impact of losses in visual acuity when presenting admixture procedures, medication self-administration, reading an EID, or securing administration set connections.

POLICY

Patient education is a process that includes assessing the learner, developing a teaching plan based on assessment results, implementing the teaching plan, and evaluating results. The patient shall be provided with information on all aspects of his or her care in a manner that he or she can understand.

PROCEDURE

1. Verify patient's identity.
2. Obtain and review physician's or legally authorized prescriber's order or treatment plan.
3. Provide privacy.
4. Prior to initiating infusion therapy, explain the procedure, its purpose, and potential side effects in sufficient detail for patient and caregiver to understand.
5. Provide written educational materials or audiovisual media to the patient and caregiver to supplement verbal explanations. Allow time for the patient and caregiver to ask questions regarding therapy.
6. Assess the patient's level of comprehension of the intended therapy and educate accordingly.
7. Document patient's knowledge deficit and readiness to learn; learning objectives; implementation of teaching plan; demonstrated skills; patient response to teaching; and an evaluation of the overall process, actions, and results of patient education in the patient's medical record.
8. For homebound patients who perform self-care, establish a comprehensive education program based on:
   - Patient's and caregiver's physical and cognitive capabilities.
   - Return demonstrations of emergency preparedness.
   - Continued access to healthcare personnel.
   - Suitability of the home environment for infusion therapy.

- Education and support of family and significant others.
- Introduction and description of involved agencies' roles and responsibilities.
- Record keeping or charting required of the patient and caregivers.
- Proper use, care, storage, and disposal of all products and equipment used in the patient's treatment.

Care Planning

CONSIDERATIONS FOR THE OLDER ADULT

The nursing care plan must address both the special needs of the patient as an individual, and his or her needs as an older adult.

The care plan should be clearly documented, detailing short- and long-term infusion care goals and objectives including any specific problems, recommendations, and time frame for goal achievement. The nurse must ensure that the plan of care takes into consideration the special needs of the older adult, including any impaired cardiac, hepatic or renal functioning, which may lead to poor tissue perfusion, impaired drug metabolism, and excretion.

POLICY

A nursing care plan shall be established for each patient receiving infusion therapy. Regardless of practice setting, elements of the nursing process, which include assessment, diagnosis, plan, implementation, and evaluation, shall be used in care planning. Care planning is a collaborative, interdisciplinary process that includes the patient, family, or other caregiver, and the healthcare team. The care plan is a dynamic tool that changes as outcomes are explored and is intended to help the patient achieve an optimum level of functioning and health.

PROCEDURE

1. Verify patient's identity.

2. Obtain and review physician's order or treatment plan.

3. Using information obtained during the patient assessment and the patient's treatment plan, develop the care plan utilizing the nursing process. Ensure that the plan of care takes into consideration the special needs of the older adult.

4. Develop goals and outcomes that are realistic and measurable. Care plan development should include attention to psychosocial support, interventions, length of therapy, mode of therapy, anticipated patient outcomes, and environment.

5. Inform the patient of the care plan and involve the patient in establishing mutually acceptable healthcare goals.

6. Document the care plan in the format established by the organization and place in the patient's medical record.

7. Review, revise, and update the care plan when there is a change in the older adult's status, needs, or physician's order, or at the frequency established by the organization, regulatory, or accrediting agency.

Discharge Planning

CONSIDERATIONS FOR THE OLDER ADULT

Several factors must be considered when planning for discharge, including the environment to which the older adult will be discharged, the ability of the older adult to participate in infusion self-care activities, and the availability and capability of a caregiver or healthcare provider to manage infusion therapy.

If the older adult is being transferred to another facility, it is especially important that the infusion needs are clearly conveyed to caregivers at the facility, including such information as:

- Existing vascular access device and location.
- Expected care regimen(s).
- Dosage and time of the most recent parenteral administrations.
- Complete list of infusion medications or solutions prescribed and administered.
- Any unusual reactions and other complications related to prescribed infusion therapy.

POLICY

The discharge planning process shall be initiated when the patient begins infusion therapy and shall continue throughout the intended therapy plan. It should not be delayed until the day of discharge.

PROCEDURE

1. Verify patient's identity.

2. Begin discharge planning when the duration of therapy is determined; discuss with patient and family.

3. Follow up on discussion with patient and family regarding discontinuation of therapy, post-discharge plans, and any follow-up care or services.

4. Coordinate with appropriate agencies any post-discharge services ordered by the physician.

5. Complete a written report evaluating the course of therapy and summarizing the discharge instructions for the patient. Send a copy to the physician and other members of the healthcare team as appropriate.

6. Document in the patient's permanent medical record.

Hand Hygiene and Infection Control

CONSIDERATIONS FOR THE OLDER ADULT

Diagnostic and therapeutic procedures can increase the patient's risk of acquiring an infection. For the older adult, this risk is augmented by age-related body system changes in functioning that impact the immune system.

The older adult may present with or develop an infection without the usual signs and symptoms. The older adult may experience a decreased basal metabolic rate and core temperature. Fever may be absent or delayed in its onset, and may be further masked by the use of antiinflammatory medications.

When teaching hand hygiene for infusion self-care to the older adult, it is important to take into consideration the patient's physical ability to stand in front of a sink, any need for ambulatory aids such as a cane or walker, skin sensitivity to waterless antiseptic products, and any cognitive impairments that may affect the ability to follow the correct sequencing of steps.

POLICY

Hand hygiene is a critically important infection control practice. When provision for hand hygiene facilities is not feasible, the organization must provide antiseptic hand cleanser or waterless antiseptic products, clean cloth or paper towels, or antiseptic towelettes.

Wash hands before and after performing patient care procedures, before donning and after removing gloves.

PROCEDURE

1. Remove jewelry.
2. Dispense soap or antiseptic solution into cupped hands and use continuously running water. (Note: Use dispensers for soap or antiseptic solution.)
3. Thoroughly cleanse the palms and backs of both hands.
4. Avoid splashing that may cause contamination of clothing and other skin surfaces.
5. Rinse hands thoroughly under running water.
6. Use clean paper towel to dry hands. Do not wave hands or blow on skin to dry.
7. Turn off faucet using same paper towel.

When Running Water Is Not Available:

1. Remove jewelry.
2. Dispense approximately 5 ml of waterless product into cupped hands.
3. Use friction over all surfaces of both hands and rub vigorously until dry (approximately 15 seconds).
4. Do not rinse with water or towel dry.
5. Wash hands with soap or antiseptic solution and water as soon as possible.

Documentation

CONSIDERATIONS FOR THE OLDER ADULT

Documentation is an important component of all aspects of patient care. Documentation serves as a confidential communication tool between all members of the healthcare team, provides a record of patient care, and indicates prescribed and implemented therapies and treatments, interventions, and outcomes.

When caring for the older adult, it is especially important to document physical and cognitive functioning or deficits, as well as patient concerns that can impact infusion-related decision-making. Documentation that accurately reflects the older adult's functioning facilitates selection of the appropriate equipment to ensure continuation of the infusion prescription post-discharge.

The nurse should document any special needs of the older adult and how they were addressed. Documentation should include how family and caregiver concerns and educational needs were met.

POLICY

Each patient receiving infusion therapy shall have a medical record. A medical record shall contain sufficient information to identify infusion procedures, prescribed treatments, complications, nursing interventions, and patient outcomes. Entries in the patient's medical record shall be factual, accurate, and legible. The record must be easily retrievable and accessible to healthcare professionals involved in the patient's care. The organization shall determine the forms, method of documentation, storage, and retention requirements of the patient's medical record.

PROCEDURE

Establish a medical record for the patient receiving infusion therapy.

A. Information to be included

To record general information, document the following in the patient's medical record:

1. Evidence that the prescribed treatment was administered
2. Evidence of initial and ongoing patient assessment, medication profile, care plan, nursing intervention, and monitoring
3. Infusion therapy procedures, complications, interventions, and patient outcomes
4. Communication among interdisciplinary healthcare professionals involved in the patient's care
5. When documenting patient education, include information that was conveyed as well as demonstrated skills, return demonstrations by the patient or caregiver, and the patient's and caregiver's overall response to teaching.
6. Evidence of the patient's and caregiver's comprehension of prescribed therapy and ability to participate in care
7. Discharge notes, summary, and instructions
8. Statistical data

To record infusion therapy, document the following:

1. Assessment, initiation, monitoring, complications, and termination of the prescribed therapy
2. Vascular access device (VAD) type, brand, gauge, and length; insertion site and condition; date and time of insertion
3. Identify (name and title) of individual inserting VAD
4. Radiological confirmation of location of catheter tip, as appropriate
5. Parenteral therapy administered
6. Equipment or device used
7. Number of venipuncture attempts
8. Use of any prescribed local anesthetic, with type and volume

To record infiltration or extravasation, document the following:

1. Volume infused
2. Date and time
3. Adverse reaction first noted
4. Interventions
5. Type, volume, and method of administration of an antidote
6. Patient complaints
7. Patient's response to intervention(s)

When removing a VAD, document the following:

1. Reason for removal: routine site rotation, discharge, or complication (including lack of blood return, positional problems, or catheter malfunction)
2. Date, time, and initials of individual removing the device
3. Description of catheter, including length
4. How removed and patient's response
5. Length of time pressure applied to site
6. Type of dressing
7. Use of antimicrobial ointment, if any
8. Patient restrictions following removal
9. Post-removal complications such as pain, phlebitis, extravasation, discharge (color, amount, odor), infection (indicating any cultures taken with results if available)
10. Communication with physician or other members of the healthcare team
11. Continuance of ongoing monitoring
    • Discontinuation of therapy
    • Patient outcome of therapy
12. Laboratory specimens collected at initiation or discontinuation of therapy

B. Guidelines for recording documentation

Document entries in patient's medical record using the following guidelines:

1. Use abbreviations and forms approved by the organization

2. If an error is made while documenting an entry, draw a line across the error and write "mistaken entry" in a way that it does not obscure the original entry; do not use correction fluid or erasures on the patient's medical record.

3. Use only permanent ink, preferably blue or black or as determined by the organization.

4. Sign all entries with full name and credentials or title of individual making entry; use of initials shall be determined by the organization.

C. Storage of the patient's permanent medical record

Store the patient's medical record:

1. In a location that affords convenient retrieval yet maintains confidentiality.

2. As hard documents, computer tapes, or microfiche.

3. In a safe environment that is protected from fires, tampering, and theft.

D. Retrieving and discarding medical records

Retain the patient's medical record for the appropriate amount of time.

1. For adults, retain patient's medical record for a minimum of seven years following last date of service, except where state regulations require retention for a longer period of time.

2. Discard medical records past the required retention time by shredding; keep written verification of date of destruction on file or as determined by the organization.

E. Confidentiality

Medical records are to remain confidential.

1. Only the patient, and individuals or regulatory agencies approved by the organization can access, make entries in, or review patient's medical record.

2. Duplication of patient's medical record will be done only upon proof of release from patient.

F. Electronic medical record

Electronic medical records can facilitate data collection for research purposes through the anonymous transfer of data to research databases via computer programs.

1. Use of electronic medical records shall be determined by the organization.

2. Provide education and training of staff using the information system.

3. Electronic key or signature password provided to users must be kept confidential, and should be changed often.

4. Provision of back-up system for documentation must be established by the organization.

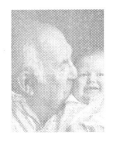

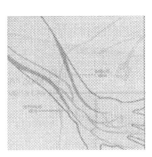

3.

Infusion Equipment

Armboards and Restraints*

CONSIDERATIONS FOR THE OLDER ADULT

Armboards are typically used to support areas of flexion when a VAD is in place.

Caution is recommended when applying the armboard to the older adult's hand or wrist area when there is evidence of arthritic joint changes. While positioning the hand or wrist in a functional position is necessary, extra padding under taping surfaces may be required to prevent joint stiffness and discomfort.

A soft restraint may be required for older adults who might otherwise accidentally dislodge a VAD. The restraint should not be applied so tightly that the patient's circulation, infusate flow, or securement of the catheter is compromised.

Collaborative efforts should be made with interdisciplinary team members to develop a plan of care that would prevent patients' attempts to remove the VAD while avoiding the use of restraints. Use the least restrictive restraining device as possible.

The older adult must be checked frequently and the restraint or armboard removed at regular intervals to allow full range of motion and circulation assessment. Reinforcement of education processes should be continued to prevent accidental dislodgment and self-injury. If there is an armboard in place, the restraint should be placed around the armboard, rather than the wrist or arm.

Armboards may be considered a form of restraint: check with organizational policy for restraint use; restraint may require a physician's order.

POLICY

Armboards or restraints are used to immobilize the affected extremity and maintain correct catheter placement in order to minimize device movement. Armboards or restraints should be used when:

1. Infusions are initiated on uncooperative or disoriented patients.
2. The catheter is inserted in the dorsum of the hand or in an area of joint flexion.
3. Skin integrity has been comprised due to accidental tearing, excessive bruising or dermal infections.

PROCEDURE

Read and follow manufacturer's guidelines for use of armboards or restraints.

1. Use armboards that are padded and conform to extremity shape and length.
2. If possible, use disposable units. If armboards or restraints are reusable, disinfect between patient use.
3. When applying armboards or restraints, assess and monitor for the following:
   • Functional position of extremity to preserve maximal function
   • Extremity or area for circulatory perfusion
   • Visibility of the infusion site
   • Signs of pending nerve or muscle impingement or damage
   • Patient comfort and daily hygiene
4. The patient should be instructed to move other joints (ie, fingers, shoulder) of the extremity to improve circulation and prevent stiffening.

5. Tape should be kept to a minimum on the skin. Tape used to apply the armboard can be backed with strips of gauze or tape to prevent skin damage.

6. It is sometimes helpful to cover the VAD lest it become a source of curiosity for the older adult who may not be fully aware of its purpose. However, nothing should be wrapped around the extremity that might impede circulation, is difficult to remove, or would make observation of the catheter-skin junction difficult.

7. Apply restraint to armboard, not to patient's arm.

8. Do not use roller bandage to restrain or keep catheter in place; it may impede circulation and does not allow for visual inspection of catheter insertion site.

9. Remove armboards or restraints at a frequency established by the organization.

EQUIPMENT
- Armboard
- Restraints

IV Poles

CONSIDERATIONS FOR THE OLDER ADULT

IV poles are not meant to be ambulatory aids and the nurse should instruct the older adult not to use them as such. IV poles must be serviced regularly to ensure that they move easily and are not a safety hazard due to sticking or locking of the wheels. If an ambulatory aid, such as a walker, is required, it is best if the pole is an integral part of the aid. Stationary IV poles are ideal for those older adults confined to bed or who are receiving intermittent infusions.

IV poles should have:
- A wide base and low center of gravity to avoid tipping.
- Wheels that move freely for ease of mobility.
- Adjustable hang height.

An infusion control device, if required, should be mounted below the adjustment area to avoid tipping.

POLICY

IV poles permit the hanging of infusate containers at appropriate heights to facilitate solution and medication delivery. Ambulatory IV poles allow for independence while ambulating and performing ADLs for older adults receiving infusion therapy.

PROCEDURE

Instruct the older adult
1. Not to use the IV pole as a walking aid.
2. To avoid carpeted areas.
3. Not to hang personal items on pole.
4. To keep floor free of obstacles.
5. To avoid stairs.

Equipment

IV pole: ambulatory or stationary

Infusion and Flow Control Devices

CONSIDERATIONS FOR THE OLDER ADULT

Control of infusion rates in the older adult is an especially important consideration. Older adults are very sensitive to rapid fluctuations in circulating volumes. Changes in cardiac and renal function that occur with aging and certain disease states require careful monitoring and titration of parenteral fluid volume delivery.

Patient education should be enforced and manufactured safety mechanisms employed when using infusion control devices. If the older adult appears confused or disoriented, precaution should be taken to avoid any inadvertent manipulation of the flow control mechanism. Lock-out, anti-free flow and other safety features should be engaged to prevent the inadvertent delivery of a bolus of parenteral fluids.

Some of these devices can be quite heavy and must be attached to an ambulatory IV pole in order for the older adult to maintain independence. Educating the older adult and caregiver(s) will help to avoid safety hazards associated with flow control devices. The device should be positioned below the adjustment cuff to prevent tipping. The patient must not use the pole as an ambulatory aid, and may require assistance in the home setting. (see Policy and Procedure: IV Poles)

POLICY

Infusion control devices assist in regulating the administration rate of parenteral solutions or medications. When using these devices, consideration shall be given to patient's age and condition, prescribed therapy, and setting where the therapy is delivered. The nurse is responsible for the use of infusion control devices and should be knowledgeable regarding the following:

1. Indications for use

2. Mechanical operation including demonstrated competency

3. Troubleshooting

4. Pounds per square inch (PSI) rating

PROCEDURE

Mechanical Flow Control Devices

Mechanical infusion control devices are compact devices that use either a balloon or spring mechanism to regulate administration of prescribed therapy.

1. Follow manufacturer's guidelines for the use of mechanical infusion control devices.

Electronic Flow Control Devices

Electronic infusion control devices (EIDs) are powered by internal battery or alternating current and are used to regulate administration of prescribed therapy.

1. Follow manufacturer's guidelines for the use of EIDs.

2. Select EID with safety features such as:
   • Audible alarm
   • Battery life and operation
   • Anti-free flow mechanism
   • Accuracy of delivery

- Drug calculation
- In-line pressure monitoring
- Adjustable occlusion pressure levels
- Antitampering mechanism

Controllers (gravity-activated):

Controllers are EIDs that generate flow by gravity and are capable of either drop counting or volumetric delivery. They can be safely used to regulate or administer

1. Vesicants.
2. Infusion via central vascular access devices (CVADs).
3. Infusion for neonatal and pediatric patients.
4. Infusion for older adults.
5. Infusion for oncology patients.

Pumps (positive pressure-activated):

Pumps are EIDs that generate flow under positive pressure and are used to regulate or administer

1. Arterial infusions.
2. High acuity therapies such as parenteral nutrition (PN) and inotropic therapies.
3. Pain management.
4. Home infusions.

Maintenance of Infusion Control Devices

1. Establish the frequency and mechanism for performing and documenting routine and preventative infusion control device maintenance.
2. Preventative maintenance should follow the manufacturer's, Joint Commission on Accreditation of Healthcare Organization's (JCAHO), and Association for the Advancement of Medical Instrumentation's (AAMI) guidelines.

Teaching Patient or Caregiver

1. Evaluate the ability of the patient or caregiver to comprehend and implement the use of infusion control devices.
2. Instruct patient or caregiver on
   - How to wear pump.
   - How to operate pump.
   - How to care for pump.
   - How to troubleshoot technical problems.
3. Document successful education and return demonstration of the infusion control device by the patient or caregiver.

EQUIPMENT

Mechanical Infusion Device (MID)

- Elastomere balloon: used primarily for the delivery of antiinfective agents and other small-volume, intermittent parenteral therapies
- Syringe piston: used primarily for the delivery of antiinfective agents
- Batteries, if appropriate

Electronic Infusion Device (EID)

1. Controllers (gravity-activated)
2. Pumps (positive pressure-activated)
3. Ambulatory infusion
4. Multi- and dual-channel
5. Patient-controlled analgesia
6. Peristaltic
7. Pulsatile
8. Syringe
9. Volumetric
10. Batteries, if appropriate

Add-on Devices

CONSIDERATIONS FOR THE OLDER ADULT

Add-on devices are intended to provide additional system access points, facilitate administration of multiple therapies, and prevent selected infusion-related complications. For the older adult's safety, these devices should be of a Leur-Lok™ design so that they attach securely, minimizing the possibility of accidental set separation or disconnection. Add-on devices will also facilitate minimization of invasive procedures for the older adult, potentially preserving peripheral vascular access for future therapies.

POLICY

When an integral in-line system is unavailable, add-on devices shall be used to achieve the prescribed therapy.

Add-on Devices:

1. Must be attached aseptically using Leur-Lok™ connection.

2. Should be primed when the administration set is primed.

3. Should be changed at established intervals, immediately upon suspected contamination or break in integrity, with each administration set change, and when the device to which it is attached is changed.

PROCEDURE

Follow manufacturer's guidelines for the use of add-on devices.

Add-On Device Change

1. Wash hands.

2. Don gloves.

3. Prepare add-on device according to manufacturer's guidelines.

4. Purge air from device by flushing with appropriate solution or infusate.

5. Aseptically remove expended add-on device.

6. Disinfect site connection with antiseptic solution.

7. Attach new sterile add-on device to administration set adapter or catheter hub using Leur-Lok™ connector to ensure connections are tight and secure.

8. Resume therapy as prescribed.

9. Discard expended supplies in appropriate receptacles.

10. Remove gloves.

11. Wash hands.

12. Document procedure in patient's medical record.

EQUIPMENT
General

- Gloves
- Receptacle for expended materials
- Alcohol pads or wipes
- Appropriate device flush solution

<u>Types of Add-on Devices</u>

- Catheter cap
- Extension loop
- Extension set
- Blood filter
- Add-on filter
- Injection/access port or cap
- Manifold set
- Microbore extension tubing
- Blunt cannula of needleless system
- Stopcock
- Administration set

Tourniquets

Considerations for the Older Adult

Due to friability of aging skin, the time and tension the tourniquet is applied should be limited to avoid inadvertent bruising and skin tears. Venous distention may take longer and tapping the area over the vein and intended venipuncture site may cause accidental bruising. If the tourniquet is too tight or is in place for an extended period of time, the vein may become overly distended and may be damaged during venipuncture.

Older adults who are disoriented may become more so during tourniquet application time, therefore, tourniquets should not be applied for longer than two to three minutes. Calm reinforcement and continuous education should alleviate the older adult's anxiety during the procedure. The tourniquet should lie flat against the skin or over clothing for additional comfort. The patient should never be left with the tourniquet in place, and it should be removed while preparing equipment for venipuncture. The tourniquet should be single-use and latex-free.

POLICY

Use of a tourniquet is required to impede venous (not arterial) flow and promote venous distention for accessing the vein.

PROCEDURE

1. Follow manufacturer's guidelines for use of tourniquets.
2. Clear extremity of clothing and bedding.
3. Fasten tourniquet at least 4 to 8 inches above intended catheter insertion site to dilate vein.
4. Place tourniquet over clothing to prevent accidental skin pinching and tearing.
5. Observe the older adult for
   • disruptions in skin integrity.
   • subcutaneous bleeding (indicator of prolonged tourniquet time).
   • worsening of existing complications such as bruising and hematoma, seeping of fluids.
6. Allow vein to fill with blood.
7. Remove tourniquet promptly at conclusion of assessment or venipuncture procedure to prevent circulatory impairment.
8. Discard tourniquet at completion of procedure.

EQUIPMENT

Tourniquet, single-use

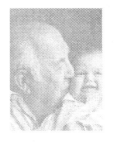

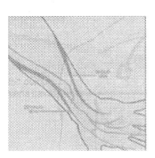

4.

Site Selection and Device Placement

Site Selection

CONSIDERATIONS FOR THE OLDER ADULT

Due to loss of subcutaneous fat and thinning of the skin in the older adult, placement of a VAD can be challenging. Lack of supporting tissues may make catheter insertion and securement more difficult, while increasing the potential risk for bruising, phlebitis, and infiltration. The nurse should select areas with more subcutaneous tissue and skeletal support for better device stabilization, keeping in mind the need to conserve peripheral access for future therapy.

Length and type of treatment must be taken into consideration when selecting potential sites. If the older adult is independent, it is important for him or her to continue these activities. An insertion site that allows for use of the hands and does not restrict range of motion is ideal.

Patient handedness is an important consideration. It is acceptable for the older adult to have input as to where the catheter will be placed, for example, in the nondominant arm. Many older adults have had previous experience with infusion therapy and can indicate what has and has not worked for them in the past. If the older adult must use an ambulatory aid to maintain independence, determine the side on which the aid will be used. It is important to avoid VAD placement in the hands and areas of flexion if possible. For the less mobile patient, consider using the extremity that most easily allows access to the bathroom or commode to minimize inadvertent catheter dislodgment or entanglement in administration set tubing.

POLICY

Vein selected for cannulation shall accommodate gauge and length of the catheter. Site selected is based on

1. Patient's condition, age, and diagnosis.
2. Vein condition, size and location.
3. Type and duration of prescribed therapy.
4. Patient's infusion history, and patient's choice of location as appropriate.

PROCEDURE

1. Site Selection for Peripheral-Short Catheter
   - Assess patient's upper extremities. (Note: Avoid using lower extremity veins in adults.)
   - Place patient in comfortable supine position
2. Assess appropriate veins on both dorsal and ventral surfaces.
   - Metacarpal
   - Cephalic
   - Basilic
   - Median cubital
3. Select the most distal site for peripheral-short catheter placement.
   - Select sites that are proximal to previous cannulation sites.
   - Avoid areas of flexion, existing phlebitis, bruises, or previous areas of infiltration.
   - Avoid arms with: compromised circulation; post-mastectomy or post-axillary node dissection; and fistulated extremities.

4. Assess availability of acceptable veins by applying tourniquet 4 to 8 inches proximal to intended venipuncture site.
   - Palpate extremity distal to tourniquet to assess vein condition and visually inspect skin integrity.
   - Palpate to differentiate arteries from veins.
   - If unable to palpate vein, instruct patient to open and close fist several times; apply warm heat to extremity for approximately 15 minutes to promote vein relaxation and dilation if necessary.
5. Select catheter insertion site.
6. Remove tourniquet.

Site Selection for Midline Catheter (ML)

1. Assess patient's upper extremities.
   - Place patient in comfortable supine position.
2. Assess antecubital fossa for veins appropriate for ML placement.
   - Cephalic
   - Basilic
   - Median cubital
3. Select appropriate site.
   - Avoid arms with: compromised circulation; post-mastectomy or post-axillary node dissection; and fistulated extremities.
4. Assess availability of acceptable veins by applying tourniquet approximately 4 inches proximal to antecubital fossa.
   - Palpate antecubital sites to assess vein condition and visually inspect skin integrity.
   - Palpate to differentiate arteries from veins.
   - If unable to adequately palpate vein, instruct patient to open and close fist several times; apply warm heat to extremity for approximately 15 minutes to promote vein relaxation and dilation if necessary.
5. Select catheter insertion site.
6. Remove tourniquet.

Site Selection for Peripherally Inserted Central Catheter (PICC)

1. Assess possible access to intended venous pathway including upper extremities and chest.
   - Place patient in comfortable supine position.
2. Assess antecubital fossa for veins appropriate for PICC placement.
   - Cephalic
   - Basilic
   - Median cubital
3. Select appropriate site.
   - Avoid arms with: compromised circulation; post-mastectomy or post-axillary node dissection; and fistulated extremities.
4. Assess availability of acceptable veins by applying tourniquet approximately 4 inches proximal to antecubital fossa.
   - Palpate antecubital sites to assess vein condition and visually inspect skin integrity.
   - Palpate to differentiate arteries from veins.

- If unable to adequately palpate vein, instruct patient to open and close fist several times; apply warm heat to extremity for approximately 15 minutes to promote vein relaxation and dilation if necessary.

5. Select catheter insertion site.

6. Remove tourniquet.

Site Selection for Central Catheter

With the exception of PICCs, site selection and insertion of a CVAD is considered a medical act.

Post-Site Selection

1. Proceed with VAD insertion, if possible.

2. Document procedure in patient's medical record.

EQUIPMENT

Tourniquet, single-use

Catheter Selection

CONSIDERATIONS FOR THE OLDER ADULT

Thickening and stiffening of vascular structures and other cardiovascular changes associated with the older adult can make catheter insertion and placement more difficult.

The nurse should select the smallest gauge catheter that will deliver the prescribed therapy, allowing for optimum blood flow around the catheter and hemodilution of the infusate. For most short-term therapies, a 22 or 24 gauge peripheral-short catheter is adequate. Larger gauge catheters can be used for transfusion of blood products (20 or 22 gauge) or large volume infusions that must be given quickly (18 or 20 gauge). Some therapies are best delivered by a CVAD.

POLICY

The selected VAD shall be radiopaque. The nurse should select the smallest gauge and shortest length to accommodate the prescribed therapy.

PROCEDURE

Selecting a peripheral-short catheter

1. Properties of a selected VAD
   - Radiopaque
   - Constructed of material that will decrease thrombogenicity and promote patient safety
   - Can be inserted and cared for by available qualified personnel
   - Cost-effective (ie, consider difficulty and time required to monitor or replace the device)
   - Smallest gauge catheter to accommodate the prescribed therapy (see Appendix 2)
2. Winged steel infusion set should be used only for single dose:
   - Short infusions of 1 to 4 hours in duration
   - Should not be used for continuous therapy

Selecting a midline catheter (ML)

1. Patients appropriate for ML access
   - May require frequent VAD restarts secondary to infusion prescription.
   - May have limited peripheral access.
   - May receive therapies via MLs including those indicated as appropriate for peripheral-short catheters.
2. Device selected for ML access should be
   - Radiopaque.
   - Designed specifically for ML access.
   - Long enough to accommodate tip placement without altering tip integrity.

Selecting a peripherally inserted central catheter (PICC):

1. Patients appropriate for PICC access
   - May require frequent VAD restarts secondary to infusion prescriptions.
   - May have limited peripheral access.
   - Are on long-term or chronic infusion therapy, greater than 2 weeks.
   - May have preexisting conditions prohibiting central catheter insertion via jugular or subclavian routes.

2. Therapies that may require PICC access include administration of
   - Parenteral nutrition with dextrose concentration greater than 10% or amino acid concentrations greater than 5%.
   - Continuous infusion of vesicant medications.
   - Therapies with extreme variation in osmolarity or pH.
   - Inotropic therapies.
   - Long-term (greater than 2 weeks) therapies including antiinfective therapy and hydration therapy.
   - Parenteral pain management.
3. Device selected for PICC access should be
   - Radiopaque.
   - Designed specifically for peripheral access.
   - Long enough to accommodate tip placement in vena cava without alteration of tip integrity; however, when tip alteration may be required, follow manufacturer's recommendations.

EQUIPMENT
General
- Gloves
- Tourniquet
- Measuring tape
- Receptacle for expended waste

Catheter
- Peripheral-short catheter
- Winged steel infusion set
- ML
- PICC
- Equipment-specific start tray

Local Anesthesia

Considerations for the Older Adult

Administration of local anesthesia may be an option for those older adults who startle easily during venipuncture. Because there is less supportive underlying tissue in the older adult, care must be taken not to nick and damage the vein or inadvertently administer the anesthetic intravascularly. It is important to assess each patient individually. Additionally, the patient's history of allergies must be taken into consideration as well as any previous experience with catheter insertions. Allow transdermal anesthetics time to produce desired results. Intradermal anesthesia, which produces a more immediate anesthetic effect, can potentially obscure the vein making venous palpation and venipuncture more difficult.

POLICY

Anesthesia shall be used to provide a localized effect during venipuncture procedures. A physician's or legally authorized prescriber's verbal or written order is required. The type of local anesthesia administered before catheter insertion is determined by the organization and may include

- Transdermal analgesic cream.
- Iontopheresis of lidocaine hydrochloride 2% with epinephrine 1:100,000 topical solution.
- Intradermal injection of lidocaine hydrochloride 1% solution.

PROCEDURE

Prior to Beginning Procedure

1. Wash hands.
2. Don gloves.
3. Use aseptic technique and observe Standard Precautions throughout procedure.

Use of Transdermal (Topical) Analgesic Cream

1. Follow manufacturer's guidelines for analgesia cream application.
2. Assess and select intended venipuncture site.
3. Cleanse area with antiinfective soap and water if necessary.
4. Disinfect site with alcohol and allow it to dry.
5. Apply layer of transdermal analgesia cream to intended venipuncture site.
6. Cover analgesia cream with transparent semipermeable membrane (TSM) dressing material and leave in place as directed by manufacturer.
7. Remove dressing material and remaining transdermal cream.
8. Disinfect site and allow it to dry.

Use of Iontopheresis

1. Follow manufacturer's guidelines for anesthesia application.

Use of Injectable (Intradermal) Anesthetic

1. Follow manufacturer's guidelines for intradermal anesthesia injections.
2. Disinfect site and allow it to dry.

3. Draw 0.3 cc of injectable anesthetic medication into 1-ml (Tuberculin) syringe.

4. With needle bevel up, gently insert needle intradermally adjacent to intended venipuncture site.

5. Aspirate to confirm negative blood return.

6. Inject 0.1 cc to 0.3 cc anesthetic to form wheal.

7. Remove needle and discard syringe in appropriate sharps container.

Post-Local Anesthesia Application

1. Monitor patient response.

2. Discard used supplies in appropriate receptacles.

3. Remove gloves.

4. Wash hands.

5. Document procedure in patient's medical record.

EQUIPMENT

General Supplies

- Gloves
- Sharps container
- Receptacle for expended waste

Topical Anesthesia

- Transdermal (topical) analgesic cream
- Occlusive TSM dressing
- Single-use alcohol swab or gauze pad(s)
- Gauze pads

Injectable Anesthesia

- Intradermal (injectable) anesthetic: Lidocaine hydrochloride 1% solution
- Single-use alcohol swab or gauze pad(s)
- 1-ml (Tuberculin) syringe
- Gauze pads

Iontopheresis

- Equipment supplied by manufacturer, with guidelines for administration

Insertion Site Preparation

CONSIDERATIONS FOR THE OLDER ADULT

Alcohol preparations can cause stinging and irritation, adding to the older adult's discomfort. Too much alcohol can dry already compromised skin. An older adult will be less likely to cooperate with venipuncture procedures if he or she experiences pain at this early stage. Be aware that, although antiseptic agents should be applied with friction, irritated skin may become more damaged, causing further distress and discomfort for the older adult.

POLICY

Catheter insertion site shall be aseptically cleansed with antiseptic solution prior to catheter placement.

PROCEDURE

Preparing Access Site for Disinfection

1. Wash hands.
2. Don gloves.
3. Wash intended venipuncture site with antiinfective soap and water if necessary.
4. Remove excess hair from insertion site with disposable clippers or scissors if necessary.
5. Administer local anesthesia if necessary.

Disinfecting Access Site

1. Select a single-dose antiseptic agent to disinfect insertion site.
2. Do not disinfect site with aqueous benzalkonium-like compounds or hexachlorophene.
3. Recommended agents include:
   - Chlorhexidine
   - 10% povidone-iodine
   - Alcohol
   - 2% tincture of iodine
4. Cleanse site using antiseptic agent according to manufacturer's recommendations for product use.
   - Allow antiseptic agent to air dry (do not blow or blot dry).
   - If using povidone-iodine as the primary antiseptic agent, do not apply alcohol, as it will negate povidone-iodine's antimicrobial effect.
   - If using alcohol as a single agent, apply for a minimum of 30 seconds.
   - If using tincture of iodine, allow it to dry, then remove with alcohol, and allow it to dry.

Post Site Disinfection

1. Discard used supplies in appropriate receptacle.
2. Remove gloves.
3. Wash hands.
4. Document procedure in patient's medical record.

EQUIPMENT

General Supplies

- Gloves
- Single-dose antiseptic agents:
  - Chlorhexidine
  - 10% povidone-iodine
  - Alcohol
  - 2% tincture of iodine
- Waste container for disposal of expended equipment

Catheter Placement

> ### CONSIDERATIONS FOR THE OLDER ADULT
>
> In the older adult, stabilization of the vein can be difficult due to changes in under-lying tissue structures. The vein wall may be difficult to penetrate due to aging processes as well as other factors. The nurse should attempt to "anchor" the vein, distal to the intended venipuncture site. Leaving the tourniquet in place for an extended period should be avoided as it may contribute to difficult VAD penetration, traumatic bruising, and could adversely impact laboratory assay collection during catheter placement. The tourniquet should be released it as soon as possible after insertion of the VAD and positive confirmation of blood return.
>
> Catheters are to be placed according to organizational policy and manufacturer's guidelines for product use. Explanations should be reinforced with each step of the procedure so the older adult is aware of what to expect. Quietly explain the procedure as it occurs in order to enhance patient cooperation and compliance. It may be helpful to have another caregiver or family member present to reassure the older adult as to the intent and expected outcome of the procedure.

POLICY

Catheters are placed for definitive therapeutic or diagnostic indications. The nurse shall use the smallest gauge, shortest length catheter capable of accomplishing the prescribed therapy.

PROCEDURE

Prior to Beginning Procedure

1. Wash hands.
2. Don gloves.
3. Use aseptic technique and observe Standard Precautions throughout procedure.

General Procedure

1. Follow manufacturer's guidelines for catheter placement.
2. Inspect the catheter for product integrity prior to insertion.
3. Use a new device for each venipuncture attempt.
4. If unsuccessful after two attempts, request another competent nurse to assess the patient for further attempts. She or he will make the determination to proceed or consult with a physician.
5. When using a device with a stylet, never reinsert the stylet into the catheter after skin and vein penetration as it may cause inadvertent shearing, puncture or fracture of the catheter.
6. When inserting a catheter through an introducer needle, never retract the catheter through the needle as it may cause inadvertent shearing, puncture or fracture of the catheter.
7. Secure device after insertion and apply dressing.
8. Label dressing with date, time, catheter gauge and length, and inserter's initials.

Post Device Securement

1. Discard used supplies in appropriate receptacles.

2. Remove gloves.

3. Wash hands.

4. Document procedure in patient's medical record.

EQUIPMENT

General Supplies

- Gloves: sterile and nonsterile
- Personal protective equipment
- Catheter
- Infusion start kit or insertion supplies
- Sharps container
- Container for expended waste

Device Securement

CONSIDERATIONS FOR THE OLDER ADULT

VADs can be secured with sterile surgical strips, sterile tapes, sterile manufactured stabilizing devices, or sutures.

Adhesive-backed tape and securement devices can cause tearing of the older adult's fragile skin if removed improperly. Tapes and securement devices must not be placed in such a way that the catheter-skin junction or the venous pathway becomes obscured and disrupts daily site inspection.

The older adult can develop sensitivities to adhesives causing redness, itching, and rash. The resulting discomfort can lead to dislodgment of the VAD due to rubbing, scratching, and pulling at the tapes. Careful early patient assessment and confirmation of allergies or allergy history will allow the nurse to plan appropriate measures to prevent adhesive-related discomfort.

POLICY

The catheter shall be stabilized in a manner that does not interfere with assessment and monitoring of catheter-skin junction or impede delivery of the prescribed therapy.

PROCEDURE

Prior to Beginning Procedure

1. Wash hands.
2. Don gloves.
3. Use aseptic technique and observe Standard Precautions throughout procedure.

Use of Sterile Tape or Sterile Surgical Strips to Secure Device

1. Follow manufacturer's guidelines for device stabilization.
2. Cleanse catheter-skin junction with appropriate antiseptic agent, being careful not to dislodge catheter prior to use of securement device.
3. Without obscuring catheter-skin junction, secure catheter hub with sterile tape or sterile surgical strips. Do not apply tape directly to catheter-skin junction site.

Use of Sterile Manufactured Securement Device

1. Follow manufacturer's recommendations for use of securement device.
2. Cleanse catheter-skin junction with appropriate antiseptic agent, being careful not to dislodge catheter prior to use of securement device.
3. Replace manufactured securement device at the time of dressing change, and according to manufacturer's recommendations for product use.

Use of Sutures to Secure Device

1. Follow manufacturer's recommendations for device securement.
2. Cleanse catheter-skin junction with appropriate antiseptic agent(s), being careful not to dislodge catheter prior to use of securement device.
3. Only skilled medical personnel may secure catheters with sutures (per state's Nurse Practice Act).
4. Use of sutures for routine catheter stabilization is not recommended unless otherwise established by the organization.

5. If sutures become loose or are no longer intact, replace, if ordered by physician, to prevent catheter migration or catheter dislodgement; or utilize alternate stabilizing techniques (eg, sterile surgical strips, sterile manufactured securement device, sterile tapes).

Post-Device Securement

1. Discard used supplies in appropriate receptacles.

2. Remove gloves.

3. Wash hands.

4. Document procedure in patient's medical record.

EQUIPMENT

General Supplies

- Sterile gloves
- Antiseptic agents for site disinfection
- Securement devices
  - Sutures
  - Sterile tapes
  - Sterile surgical strips
  - Sterile manufactured securement devices
- Sharps container
- Expended equipment receptacle

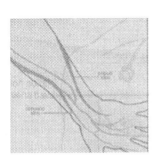

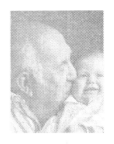

5.

Care and Maintenance

Dressing Change

> ## CONSIDERATIONS FOR THE OLDER ADULT
>
> Because of age-related changes, especially in the immune system, the older adult will be more susceptible to infectious processes. Remote infections may predispose the older adult to catheter-related blood stream infections. Changes in sensorium and cognition may predispose the older adult to accidental manipulations of the infusion catheter and dressing materials, disrupting protective care and maintenance practices such as dressing maintenance and contamination of the catheter-skin junction and administration system. Urinary incontinence and accidental separation or dislodgement of enteral feeding systems may also affect catheter dressing integrity. Extra securement measures such as additional taping and wraps that obscure the venipuncture site as protective measures will hinder daily site observations and implementation of appropriate interventions.
>
> In the older adult, skin care is of utmost importance. Unocclusive or compromised dressing materials must be changed as soon as possible. Antimicrobial cleansing agents are often very drying or irritating to the skin. The skin must be inspected with each dressing change for any adverse reaction to antiseptic solutions, adhesives, pressure areas (from catheter hubs or administration sets and add-on devices), or the macerating effects of leakage of infusates or bodily fluids from the catheter-skin junction. These are a medium for bacterial growth and their presence may necessitate more frequent dressing changes or VAD replacement.

POLICY

Sterile dressing shall be aseptically applied at initiation of vascular access, when integrity of the dressing is compromised, and at predetermined and specified time intervals.

PROCEDURE

Prior to Beginning Procedure

1. Wash hands.
2. Don clean gloves.
3. Use aseptic technique and observe Standard Precautions throughout procedure.

Gauze Dressing

Vascular access site may be covered with sterile gauze.

1. Remove expended dressing and discard in appropriate receptacle; inspect catheter-skin junction.
2. Don sterile gloves.
3. Cleanse (disinfect) area with antiseptic solution(s), and allow it to dry.
4. Aseptically position sterile gauze over catheter insertion site.
5. Seal dressing edges with sterile tapes.
6. Document date, time, catheter gauge and length, and nurse's initials on dressing margin.
7. Do not cover dressing with roller bandage.
8. Change dressing every 48 hours.
9. Change dressing immediately if integrity is compromised, or if there is drainage or moisture.

Note: When TSM is applied over gauze, it is considered a gauze dressing and must be changed every 48 hours.

Use of Transparent Semipermeable Membrane (TSM)

Vascular access site may be covered with TSM dressing.

1. Remove expended dressing and discard in appropriate receptacle; inspect catheter-skin junction.
2. Don sterile gloves.
3. Cleanse (disinfect) area with antiseptic solution(s), and allow it to dry.
4. Apply TSM according to manufacturer's recommendation.
5. Aseptically position sterile dressing over insertion site.
   - Gently smooth dressing from center toward edge.
   - Do not apply excessive tension as skin shearing may result.
6. Document date, time, catheter gauge and length, and nurse's initials on dressing margin.
7. Avoid sealing TSM dressing edges with tape.
8. Do not cover dressing with roller bandage.
9. Change dressing immediately if integrity is compromised, or if there is excessive drainage or moisture.
10. Change dressing at the following intervals:
    - For peripheral-short catheter sites: change TSM dressing at time of site rotation.
    - For catheter sites other than peripheral-short catheter sites, change TSM dressing every 3 to 7 days.

Post Site Dressing Change

1. Discard used supplies.
2. Remove gloves.
3. Wash hands.
4. Document in patient's medical record.

EQUIPMENT

General Supplies

- Nonsterile gloves
- Sterile gloves
- Antiseptic solutions
- Dressing material
- Gauze
- TSM
- Sterile tape
- Labels
- Waste receptacle for expended equipment

Note: Premade or custom-made kits or trays may contain all equipment needed for procedure.

Flushing

> ### CONSIDERATIONS FOR THE OLDER ADULT
>
> In addition to maintaining device patency, flushing serves as an infection control measure. With appropriate technique, flushing prevents the formation of an intraluminal thrombus which can serve as a nidus for bacterial growth.
>
> Use of single-dose units of flush medications will also help to prevent catheter-related infections. Flushing with preservative-free 0.9% sodium chloride, injection, is necessary before and after each intermittent infusion. Peripheral-short catheters can be "locked" using preservative-free 0.9% sodium chloride, injection. CVADs should be flushed with single-dose heparin solution (1u-100u/ml), patient condition permitting, according to manufacturer's recommendations for CVAD use.
>
> Arthritis or other musculoskeletal and neurological changes associated with disease and aging can impair manual dexterity. Syringes, prefilled by the manufacturer, can greatly enhance the older adult's or caregiver's ability to participate in self-care practices. For those who are visually impaired, color-coded or large print-labels can be supplied by the pharmacy.

POLICY

Flushing is performed to ensure and maintain patency of the VAD, and to prevent the mixing of medications and solutions that are incompatible.

Routine flushing shall be performed with the following:

- Administration of blood and blood components
- Blood sampling
- Administration of incompatible medications or solutions
- Administration of medication
- Intermittent therapy
- Conversion from continuous to intermittent infusion therapies

PROCEDURE

Prior to Beginning Procedure

1. Wash hands.
2. Don gloves.
3. Use aseptic technique and observe Standard Precautions throughout procedure.

Flushing

1. Follow manufacturer's recommendations for flushing certain VADs.
2. Disinfect catheter port with antiseptic solution.
3. If resistance or complication occurs at anytime during flushing, discontinue and notify physician.

With preservative-free 0.9% sodium chloride, injection, only

1. Flush with preservative-free 0.9% sodium chloride, injection, to maintain patency of intermittent VADs and intermittent CVADs with closed distal tip and three-position valve.
2. Connect preservative-free 0.9% sodium chloride, injection-filled syringe to catheter via insertion into prepared injection/access port.

3. Slowly aspirate until positive blood return is obtained to confirm catheter patency.

4. Slowly inject flush, maintaining positive pressure.

5. Activate extension clamping mechanism, if available.

6. Disconnect syringe from injection/access port.

With heparin only

1. Flush with heparin to maintain patency of intermittent VADs and intermittent CVADs.

2. Connect heparin-filled syringe to catheter via insertion into prepared injection/access port.

3. Slowly aspirate until positive blood return is obtained to confirm catheter patency.

4. Slowly inject flush maintaining positive pressure.

5. Activate extension clamping mechanism, if available.

6. Disconnect syringe from injection/access port.

Using the SASH (Saline-Administration-Saline-Heparin) Method

Note: Use SASH flushing procedure when heparin is used for end flushing and when heparin is not compatible with administered medications or solutions.

1. Connect first preservative-free 0.9% sodium chloride, injection-filled syringe to injection/access port.

2. Slowly aspirate until positive blood return is obtained to confirm catheter patency.

3. Flush with preservative-free 0.9% sodium chloride, injection.

4. Activate extension clamping mechanism, if available.

5. Remove syringe and discard in appropriate container.

6. Cleanse port with appropriate antiseptic solution.

7. Connect medication or solution administration set to injection/access port.

8. Administer medication or solution.

9. Activate extension clamping mechanism and disconnect medication or solution from injection/access port.

10. Cleanse injection/access port with appropriate antiseptic solution.

11. Connect second preservative-free 0.9% sodium chloride, injection-filled syringe to injection/access port.

12. Flush with preservative-free 0.9% sodium chloride, injection.

13. Activate extension clamping mechanism, if available.

14. Remove syringe and discard in appropriate container.

15. Disinfect injection/access port with antiseptic solution.

16. Connect heparin-filled syringe to injection/access port and slowly aspirate to reconfirm positive blood aspirate.

17. Slowly inject heparin flush, maintaining positive pressure.

18. Activate clamping mechanism, if available.

19. Disconnect syringe from injection/access port and discard in appropriate receptacle.

Post Flush Procedure

1. (Optional) Apply new sterile catheter adapter to port according to manufacturer's recommendations specific to needleless system in use.
2. Apply new sterile needleless adapter or catheter to administration set.
3. Monitor patient's response.
4. Discard expended supplies in appropriate receptacles.
5. Remove gloves.
6. Wash hands.
7. Document in patient's medical record.

EQUIPMENT

General Supplies

- Gloves
- Sharps container
- Receptacle for expended waste

Flushing Supplies

- Sterile injection/access port
- Flush solution(s):
    - Preservative-free 0.9% sodium chloride, injection, 10 ml
    - Heparin, 1 unit-100 unit/ml vials, 5 ml
- Syringe(s): 3, 5, and 10 ml size

Note: Premade or custom-made kits or trays may contain all equipment needed for procedure.

Administration Set and Set Change

CONSIDERATIONS FOR THE OLDER ADULT

Administration sets can pose a problem for older adults who have impaired vision, are restless in bed, or are cognitively impaired. Set tubing can become entangled in bed linen, caught on side rails or other furniture, increasing the risk for the dislodgment of the vascular access device. For those who are not confined to bed, long tubing can be a safety hazard, creating the potential for injury from tripping or falling.

Infusion rates of less than 60 ml per hour should be administered via microbore sets for accuracy of fluid delivery. Administration sets with microdrip chambers are recommended to control the administration of fluids and medications in the volume-sensitive older adult.

POLICY

Administration sets, including add-on devices and tubing, shall be changed immediately when contamination is suspected or when product integrity is compromised. Otherwise, administration sets, including add-on devices and tubing, shall be changed at established intervals depending on the type of administration and infusate.

Set Change Frequency by Administration Type (see Table 1)

1. Continuous administration-primary and secondary sets
   - If the infusate is administered continuously via primary or secondary administration set, regardless of add-on devices, change set every 72 hours.
   - The secondary set change should coincide with the primary administration set change and with the initiation of new parenteral fluids.
2. Intermittent administration-primary sets
   - If the infusate is administered intermittently, regardless of add-on devices, change set every 24 hours.

Set Change Frequency by Infusate (see Table 2)

1. Blood or blood components
   - Continuous Administration: If blood or blood component is administered continuously, regardless of add on devices, change set at the end of 4 hours.
   - Intermittent Administration: If a single unit of blood or blood component is administered, regardless of add-on devices, change set after each unit.
2. Lipid emulsions
   - Continuous Administration: If lipid emulsion units are administered continuously, regardless of add-on devices, change set every 24 hours.
   - Intermittent Administration: If a single unit of lipid emulsion is administered, regardless of add-on devices, change set after each unit.
3. Parenteral nutrition
   - Continuous Administration: If parenteral nutrition is administered continuously, regardless of add-on devices, change set every 24 hours.
   - Intermittent Administration: If parenteral nutrition is administered intermittently, regardless of add-on devices, change set every 24 hours.

PROCEDURE

Prior to Beginning Procedure

1. Wash hands.

2. Don gloves.

3. Use aseptic technique and observe Standard Precautions throughout procedure.

Administration Set Change

1. Inspect new equipment.
    - Infusate
    - Administration set (Note: Blood and blood products need separate specific administration sets)
    - Add-on devices including filters and extension tubing

2. Assemble equipment.
    - Close clamp on new administration set.
    - Attach add-on devices to administration set using Luer-Lok™ connectors.

3. Prepare infusate container.
    - Remove protective covers from administration set's spike and infusate's access port.
    - Aseptically insert spike into inverted infusate container.
    - Right and hang infusate container.

4. Prime new administration set including add-on devices.
    - Squeeze drip chamber to fill to manufacturer's mark (approximately 1/3-1/2 full).
    - Slowly open clamp to prime tubing while holding distal end of set upright, allowing filter and flow control device to hang upside-down.
    - Prime entire length of set.

5. Clamp tubing.
    - If infusion flow control device is used, leave in-line device open and clamp with add-on device.
    - If pump or controller is used, thread primed tubing through flow control device.
    - Clamp set.

6. Disconnect old administration set.
    - Clamp set.
    - If used, turn off EID.
    - Disconnect set from patient.
    - If old infusate container is still in use, invert bag and remove tubing spike; insert new administration set spike (see above).

7. If infusing into an existing VAD:
    - Clamp old administration set, clamp catheter, and disconnect from catheter hub.
    - Aseptically disinfect catheter hub.
    - Remove protective cap from distal end of set and attach to catheter hub.
    - Secure connection.
    - Unclamp catheter.
    - Discard old secondary set and infusate container.

8. Begin infusion.
    - Slowly open clamp of set to begin infusion or turn on EID.
    - Monitor drops per minute manually by counting drops, or observe EID operation to ensure proper administration rate.

Post-Set Change

1. Discard used supplies.
2. Remove gloves.
3. Wash hands.
4. Label administration set tubing.
5. Document in patient's medical record.

EQUIPMENT

General Supplies

- Gloves
- Labels
- Alcohol pads or swabs
- Receptacle for expended waste
- Tape

Infusion Administration Supplies

- Infusate
- Infusion administration set
- Add-on devices:
  - Injection/access port or cap
  - Filter
  - Manual infusion device
  - Antireflux valve
  - Manifold
  - Extension tubing
  - Stopcock
  - Needleless access cannula

Table 1: Set Change Frequency by Administration Type

Note: Change set immediately if contamination is suspected or product integrity is compromised.

Administration Type	Administration Set	Set Change Frequency
Continuous	• Primary sets • Secondary "piggyback" sets	*Standard set change interval:* • If infusate is administered continuously via primary or secondary administration set, regardless of add-on devices, change set(s) every 72 hours. (Note: Secondary "piggyback" set change should coincide with primary administration set change.)
Intermittent	• Primary sets	*Standard set change interval:* • If infusate is administered intermittently at established intervals, regardless of add-on devices, change set every 24 hours.

Source: Infusion Nurses Society. *Policies and Procedures for Infusion Nursing*, 2nd ed. Norwood, MA: Infusion Nurses Society; 2002: 105.

Table 2: Set Change Frequency by Infusate

Infusates composed of organic compounds decompose quickly. Therefore, change set, including add-on devices, more frequently than standard time intervals.

Note: Regardless of infusate, change set immediately if contamination is suspected or product integrity is compromised.

Infusate Type	Administration Type	Standard Set Change Frequency
Blood and/or Blood Components	Continuous	If blood or blood component is administered continuously, regardless of add-on devices, change set at end of 4 hours.
	Intermittent	If a single unit of blood or blood component is administered, regardless of add-on devices, change set after each unit.
Lipid Emulsions	Continuous	If lipid emulsion units are administered continuously, regardless of add-on devices, change set every 24 hours.
	Intermittent	If a single unit of lipid emulsion is administered, regardless of add-on devices, change set after each unit.
Parenteral Nutrition	Continuous	If parenteral nutrition is administered continuously, regardless of add-on devices, change set every 24 hours.
	Intermittent	If parenteral nutrition is administered intermittently, regardless of add-on devices, change set every 24 hours.

Source: Infusion Nurses Society. *Policies and Procedures for Infusion Nursing*, 2nd ed. Norwood, MA: Infusion Nurses Society; 2002: 105.

Catheter Removal

> ### CONSIDERATIONS FOR THE OLDER ADULT
> Tape and other adhesive materials used on the older adult must be removed carefully to avoid skin injury including tearing and bruising. An adhesive remover can be helpful for the process.

POLICY

A catheter shall be removed with a specific order from a physician or legally authorized prescriber when therapy is completed, during routine site rotation, when contamination or complication is suspected, or when tip location is no longer appropriate for prescribed therapy.

PROCEDURE

Prior to Beginning Procedure

1. Wash hands.

2. Don sterile gloves.

3. Use aseptic technique and observe Standard Precautions throughout procedure.

4. Educate patient as to procedure.

5. Place patient in supine position for removal of all CVADs, medical condition permitting. Patient may assume sitting or reclining position for removal of peripheral-short or ML.

Catheter Removal

1. Follow manufacturer's guidelines for catheter removal, particularly for MLs and PICCs. Do not remove tunneled and cuffed catheters or implanted ports and pumps, as it is the physician's responsibility to remove such devices. A nurse educated and competent in the removal of nontunneled, noncuffed VADs may do so per organizational policy.

2. Position patient comfortably.
   • Sitting or reclining for peripheral-short VADs or MLs.
   • Recumbent for all other peripheral VADs and CVADs

3. Discontinue administration of all infusates.

4. Remove dressing from insertion site.

5. Inspect catheter-skin junction.

6. Disinfect catheter-skin junction.

7. If appropriate, remove sutures or other catheter securement device.

8. Place first two fingers of nondominant hand lightly above catheter-skin junction site with sterile gauze pad between fingers.

9. Using gentle, even pressure, slowly retract catheter from insertion site with dominant hand while stabilizing area with nondominant hand, holding gauze. (Note: Use extreme caution when removing central nontunneled, noncuffed catheters or PICCs to prevent the occurrence of air embolism.)
   • If CVAD removal: teach patient Valsalva maneuver.
   • If the patient is unable to perform this maneuver, the dressing and any securement device(s) should be removed and, with the patient in a recumbent position and upon respiratory expiration, the catheter is removed. The nurse should immediately cover

the site with occlusive sterile gauze and apply digital pressure until hemostasis is achieved. The gauze is then replaced by an occlusive sterile dressing with an antimicrobial ointment applied directly over the exit site.

10. If resistance or complication occurs, discontinue removal and notify the physician immediately.

11. Assess integrity of removed catheter.
   • Compare length of catheter to original insertion length to ensure entire catheter is removed.

12. Dress wound exit site.
   • Apply pressure to site with sterile gauze for a minimum of 30 seconds.
   • Reapply new sterile gauze with application of approved antiseptic ointment to exit site.
   • Secure gauze to site, covering with occlusive material, ie, TSM dressing.
   • Change dressing every 24 hours until exit site is healed.

Post-Catheter Removal

1. Discard used supplies in appropriate receptacle.

2. Remove gloves.

3. Wash hands.

4. If catheter defect is noted, report to manufacturer and regulatory agencies; complete Unusual Occurrence Report as established by the organization.

5. Document procedure in patient's medical record.

EQUIPMENT

General Supplies

   • Gloves: sterile, non-sterile
   • Sharps container
   • Suture removal kit (if appropriate)
   • Measuring tape
     - Expended waste receptacle

Site Dressing

   • Antiseptic ointment
   • Dressing material:
     - Gauze
     - Transparent semipermeable membrane (TSM)
   • Tape
   • Labels

Note: Pre-made or custom-made kits or trays may contain all equipment needed for procedure.

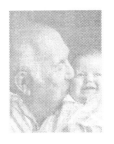

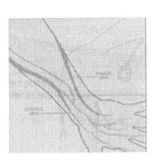

6.

Complication Management

Catheter-Related Complications

Infection

> ### CONSIDERATIONS FOR THE OLDER ADULT
>
> Cognitive and sensory deficiencies can make the older adult less reliable when reporting discomfort in early stages of catheter-related infection development. Confusion, disorientation, delirium, sleepiness and other aberrations of normal behavior may be early indicators of infection. Infection can occur locally at the venipuncture site or may be systemic. Primary infections located distant from the catheter-skin junction may also contribute to catheter-related infections and systemic infections. Patient noncompliance with care and maintenance strategies may contribute to infectious compromise. Reinforcement of patient education, especially in older adults with cognitive impairments, is necessary.

POLICY

Assessment for catheter-related infections shall be performed daily. If infections are identified, the physician shall be notified.

Catheter-related infection is a potentially life-threatening complication of infusion therapy; the infection may be local or systemic.

Local infection:

Catheter-related local infection usually occurs at the insertion site, exit site of tunneled catheters, or implanted port pocket.

Systemic infection:

Catheter-related systemic infection (sepsis) is the presence of greater than 10-15 times the colony-forming units of bacteria per ml of blood obtained through the vascular access device with no other identifiable source of infection.

PROCEDURE

Patient Assessment

1. Assess patient for signs and symptoms of catheter-related sepsis. Signs and symptoms are similar to septicemia and may be associated with febrile episode(s).
2. If patient exhibits such symptoms, include the following to assess whether or not the infection is device-related:
   - Presence of a vascular access device
   - Presence of inflammation or purulence at catheter-skin junction
   - Sudden onset of symptoms
   - Symptoms occur or increase at start of infusion or when infusion rate increases
   - Cultures confirm catheter-related infection
3. Signs and symptoms of exit site infection:
   - Tenderness
   - Erythema
   - Induration
   - Purulence within 2 cm of catheter-skin junction

4. Signs and symptoms of implanted port-pocket infection:
   - Erythema
   - Necrosis of skin over reservoir of implanted port
   - Tenderness
   - Induration
   - Purulent exudate from needle access site
   - Purulent exudate from subcutaneous pocket containing reservoir
5. Signs and symptoms of tunneled catheter track infection:
   - Erythema
   - Tenderness
   - Induration in tissues overlying catheter and greater than 2 cm from catheter exit site
6. Risk factors for catheter-related infections:
   - Dwell time
   - Catheter material, diameter, and configuration
   - Multiple manipulations of VAD due to intermittent administration of infusates
   - Catheters placed in neck or chest area
   - Catheters used for dialysis or hemodynamic monitoring
   - Use of nontunneled, noncuffed catheters
   - Compromised immune status of patient
   - Patient age
   - Presence of distant infection
   - Adequacy of nurse's competence in insertion technique

Nursing Interventions

1. To prevent catheter-related infections:
   - Observe aseptic technique and hand hygiene.
   - Inspect access site and equipment at established intervals.
   - Change administration set at established intervals.
   - Educate patient and caregiver(s) on catheter care and maintenance, complications, and preventive measures.
2. If local infection is suspected:
   - Notify physician immediately.
   - With physician's order, obtain site culture to verify presence of local infection.
   - If culture is positive, notify physician.
   - Apply topical ointment to affected area, if appropriate.
   - As ordered, apply warm compresses, if appropriate.
   - Initiate oral or parenteral antiinfective therapy as ordered.
   - If unsuccessful in treating port-pocket or tunnel track infection, VAD may need to be removed.
3. If catheter-related systemic infection is suspected:
   - Notify physician immediately.
   - Obtain blood cultures from device and from separate peripheral venipuncture site.

- Culture infusate if there is possibility of infusion-related contamination.
- Initiate parenteral antiinfectives through device if ordered.
- If unsuccessful in treating suspected catheter-related systemic infection, VAD may need to be discontinued.

Post Nursing Interventions

1. Document the following in patient's medical record:
   - Observations and patient assessment
   - Physician notification
   - Interventions taken and outcome
   - Patient's condition and response to interventions
2. Maintain statistical data on incidence of catheter-related infections, treatment, and outcome.
3. Complete Unusual Occurrence Report as required by the organization.

Catheter-Related Complications

Occlusion

CONSIDERATIONS FOR THE OLDER ADULT

Catheter occlusion is the partial or complete obstruction of a VAD preventing or limiting the infusion of solution or medication. Occlusion of the catheter can occur if blood is allowed to flow back- or reflux-into the catheter's lumen, due to improper flushing technique or infrequent monitoring of the infusion and patient's activity. Device occlusion can occur when incompatible medications are administered without flushing between delivery or due to flawed catheter dressing application.

Patient positioning is often an important factor in the prevention of catheter occlusion, especially if the catheter has been inserted near an area of flexion. The older adult may be forgetful or physically contracted. Bed clothing may become binding or constrictive as may restraints, making flow rates difficult to maintain. It is helpful to avoid VAD use in areas of flexion and to practice judicious use of armboards and restraints. The use of armboards or restraints does not take the place of frequent assessment of the patient and the infusion delivery system.

POLICY

Specific agents used to clear catheter occlusions are to be administered upon physician's order. Peripheral catheters should be removed if found to be occluded. CVADs should be treated with thrombolytic or precipitate-clearing agents when possible and after ascertainment of device integrity.

The two basic types of occlusions are:

Thrombotic occlusion

Caused by the development of a thrombus due to fibrin or coagulated blood products within or surrounding the catheter.

Non-thrombotic occlusion

Caused by mechanical obstruction such as catheter malposition or migration, drug or mineral precipitates, or lipid residue.

PROCEDURE

Patient Assessment

1. Assess patient and catheter for warning signs and symptoms of possible catheter occlusion. (see p.68 for Nursing Interventions)

Nursing Interventions

Occlusion Type	Steps to Catheter Clearance
Thrombotic Catheter Occlusion	
• Fibrin or Coagulated Blood Products	1. Notify physician immediately. 2. Obtain treatment orders for use of thrombolytic agent for catheter clearance. 3. Perform catheter clearance.
Non-Thrombotic Catheter Occlusion	
• Mechanical Obstruction	1. Notify physician immediately. 2. If catheter or administration set is kinked or clamped, unkink or unclamp catheter or set. 3. If in-line filter is clogged, replace filter. 4. If sutures securing vascular access device are constricting catheter, obtain orders to remove sutures. Reapply appropriate stabilizing device for catheter securement. 5. If noncoring needle is not in septum, remove and replace needle correctly and appropriately.
• Pinch-Off Syndrome	1. Notify physician immediately. 2. If x-ray is ordered, notify radiologist of the possibility of Pinch-Off Syndrome. 3. Further clinical intervention will depend on grade of catheter path
• Catheter Rupture	See *Policy on Embolism: Catheter*, page 72.
• Catheter Malposition or Migration	1. Notify physician immediately. 2. Reposition patient to change direction of catheter tip. 3. Inject fluid rapidly through catheter as ordered by physician. 4. Catheter may be repositioned fluoroscopically as ordered by the physician. 5. Catheter may be partially withdrawn using aseptic technique if appropriate. 6. If attempts to reposition catheter are unsuccessful, notify physician and obtain orders to remove device.
• Drug and Mineral Precipitates	1. Notify physician immediately. 2. Obtain orders for trial instillation of thrombolytics to rule out thrombotic occlusion. 3. Obtain orders to perform catheter clearance. 4. Clear catheter using hydrochloric acid, cysteine hydrochloride, sodium bicarbonate, ethanol, or sodium hydroxide as indicated.
• Lipid Residue	1. Notify physician immediately. 2. Obtain orders to clear catheter using 70% ethanol or sodium hydrochloride. 3. Perform catheter clearance.

Source: Infusion Nurses Society. *Policies and Procedures for Infusion Nursing.* 2nd edition. Norwood, MA: Infusion Nurses Society; 2002: 116.

Prevention of Catheter Occlusion

To prevent catheter occlusion:

- Flush access device.
- Promptly correct any obvious signs of mechanical obstruction.
- Use in-line air-eliminating filter.
- Monitor infusions of potential precipitate-forming solutions (ie, calcium-phosphate solutions).
- Monitor use of three-in-one parenteral nutrition admixtures.
- Avoid excessive ambient temperature fluctuations during PN administration.

Post-Nursing Intervention

1. Document the following in patient's medical record:
   - Observations and patient assessment
   - Physician notification
   - Interventions taken and outcome
   - Patient's condition and response to interventions
2. Maintain statistical data on incidence of catheter occlusions, cause, treatment, and outcome.
3. Complete Unusual Occurrence Report as established by the organization.

Catheter-Related Complications

Embolism: Catheter

CONSIDERATIONS FOR THE OLDER ADULT

Catheter embolism occurs when a piece of catheter has fractured off and travels into the vascular system creating blockage, loss of circulation, cardiac irritability, or cardiac arrest.

While there are several ways for catheter fracture to occur, it is particularly important to assess the older adult for prevention of this untoward event. The cognitively impaired older adult may manipulate unfamiliar objects in his or her immediate environment, including infusion catheters, devices and other related equipment. If a catheter becomes inadvertently dislodged, careful inspection must be made to ascertain that the device is intact, according to manufacturer's configuration and length. The older adult may not be able to adequately describe associated symptoms of catheter fracture or embolization, so careful monitoring by the nurse is necessary. The nurse should pay particular attention to patient education, encourage patient compliance, and place therapy restrictions on daily activities to promote older adult safety.

POLICY

A catheter embolus can be introduced into the circulation when

1. A through-the-needle catheter is pulled backward and then threaded forward, causing the catheter to be pierced or severed.
2. An over-the-needle catheter stylet is partially withdrawn then reinserted into the catheter.
3. A catheter ruptures or breaks after placement.
4. Excessive pressure is used when flushing the catheter causing it to fracture.
5. Catheter ruptures as a result of Pinch-Off Syndrome.

Peripheral vascular access devices shall be assessed for patency, for catheter and hub separation, or for severance upon removal. Upon removal, CVADs shall be assessed for patency, for catheter and hub separation, or for severance or fracture.

PROCEDURE

Patient Assessment

1. Assess patient for signs and symptoms of catheter embolism.
2. Severity of symptoms may depend on location of embolus.
   - Cyanosis
   - Hypotension
   - Tachycardia
   - Syncope or loss of consciousness
3. Monitor patient's vital signs.

Nursing Interventions

1. To prevent catheter embolism:
   - Inspect catheters for defects prior to use.
   - Never pull catheter back through needle when using through-the-needle catheter.
   - Never withdraw or reinsert over-the-needle catheter once it is partially or fully threaded.

- Use appropriate size syringe and technique when flushing.

2. If peripheral catheter embolism is suspected:
   - Place tourniquet above venipuncture site, tight enough so as not to occlude arterial flow; check patient's pulse at frequent intervals.
   - Place patient on strict bed rest.
   - Notify the physician immediately.
   - Monitor patient closely for signs of distress.
   - Perform interventions and treatments per physician's order.
   - Have emergency resuscitative equipment available.

3. If central vascular catheter embolism is suspected:
   - Place patient on strict bed rest.
   - Notify physician immediately.
   - Monitor patient closely for signs of distress.
   - Perform interventions and treatments as ordered.
   - If radiographic extraction of catheter embolus is necessary, educate patient on procedure.

Post Nursing Intervention

1. Document the following in patient's medical record:
   - Observations and patient assessment
   - Physician notification
   - Interventions taken and outcome
   - Patient's condition and response to interventions

2. Maintain statistical data on incidence of catheter embolism, cause, treatment, and outcome.

3. Complete Unusual Occurrence Report as established by the organization.

Catheter-Related Complications

Phlebitis

CONSIDERATIONS FOR THE OLDER ADULT

The older adult can be at particular risk for phlebitis due to alterations in the integumentary system, fluid and electrolyte imbalances, malnutrition, and other pre-existing disease processes. They are often exposed to multiple parenteral medications and solutions with chemical properties that are inherently irritating. Phlebitis can also contribute to medication error by delay of therapy administration and fluctuations in therapeutic medication levels secondary to delivery disruption.

Additionally, improper care of the VAD, prolonged or extended catheter dwell, poor insertion technique, inappropriate site selection, and underlying factors such as disease and age can all contribute to phlebitis formation.

Provide the older adult and his or her caregiver with instructions on how to recognize signs and symptoms of phlebitis, and continue to reinforce this education throughout continuation of therapy.

POLICY

Phlebitis, inflammation of the vein characterized by pain and tenderness along the course of the vein pathway, is a common complication during the administration of infusion therapy. Phlebitis may occur up to 48 hours after catheter removal. The degree of phlebitis shall be documented in the patient's medical record and the catheter removed immediately.

PROCEDURE

Patient Assessment

1. Assess patient, insertion site, and patient's extremities for signs of phlebitis.
    - Inspect insertion site frequently for signs of tenderness, redness, or inflammation.
    - Palpate skin around catheter tip to check for tenderness and vein induration.
    - Observe skin and insertion site for warmth, edema, and vein induration.
    - Assess patient regarding presence of pain, heat, stinging, burning, and discomfort at access site.
2. Consider type, pH, osmolarity, concentration, rate and volume of solution or medication infused into the affected area.
3. After removal of catheter from site, observe site for signs of post-infusion phlebitis, such as inflammation, erythema, edema, and drainage; palpate site for warmth and vein induration.
4. Document in patient's medical record.
5. When assessing for phlebitis or post-infusion phlebitis, consideration should be given to
    - Nurse's catheter insertion technique.
    - Nurse's catheter removal technique.
    - Condition and age of the patient.
    - Condition of the vein.
    - Gauge, length, and size of catheter.
    - Compatibility, type, pH, and osmolarity of solution or medication.

6. Type of filtration.
7. Measure degree of phlebitis using the **Phlebitis Scale**. The scale provides a uniform standard for measuring the degree of phlebitis.

Grade	Clinical Criteria
0	No symptoms
1	Erythema at access site with or without pain
2	Pain at access site with erythema and/or edema
3	Pain at access site with erythema and/or edema Streak formation Palpable venous cord
4	Pain at access site with erythema and/or edema Streak formation Palpable venous cord > 1 inch in length Purulent drainage

Source: Infusion Nurses Society. Infusion Nursing Standards of Practice. *J Intravenous Nurs.* 2000; 23(6S): S56.

Nursing Interventions

Once phlebitis is suspected

1. Discontinue infusion.
2. Remove catheter.
3. Disinfect venipuncture site.
4. Apply pressure at catheter removal site to achieve hemostasis.
5. Apply intermittent warm, moist heat to phlebitis site for 20-minute periods 3-4 times per day, with physician's order. (Note: Depending on cause of phlebitis, on some occasions, applications of cold compresses or ice may be more appropriate.)
6. If catheter-related infection is suspected, remove catheter aseptically and send for culture.
7. If purulent drainage is present, obtain a culture sample of drainage prior to cleaning site.
8. Notify physician regarding degree of phlebitis.

Post Nursing Intervention

1. Document in patient's medical record.
2. When inserting new catheter, do not use affected (phlebitic) arm.
   • Use opposite extremity, if possible.
   • Avoid areas of flexion.
   • Educate patient as to preventive measures as well as signs and symptoms of phlebitis development.
3. Maintain statistical data on phlebitis rates including degree, incidence, cause, and correction.

Infusion-Related Complications

Infiltration

> ### CONSIDERATIONS FOR THE OLDER ADULT
>
> Infiltration is the inadvertent administration of a nonvesicant solution or medication into surrounding tissues as a result of catheter dislodgment. Infiltration of solutions or medications could lead to impairment of functional capabilities, which could result in diminished capacities for self-care. Infiltration can also contribute to medication error by delay of therapy administration and fluctuations in therapeutic medication levels secondary to delivery disruption.
>
> Accidental dislodgment of the VAD may go unnoticed due to changes in the older adult's sensorium, less elastic tissues, and other conditions. Diminished responses to noxious stimuli may delay verbalized complaints. Older adults tend not to report discomfort and pain as frequently as younger patients. Such patients can be accurately assessed when prompted more frequently.
>
> Older adults may feel they are expected to tolerate some level of pain. Expression of discomfort may be considered a weakness, he or she may fear being viewed as "difficult," or may fear that there is a serious reason for the pain such as disease progression and imminent death.

POLICY

Nurses must be knowledgeable regarding the signs and symptoms of infiltration and shall initiate corrective measures at the onset of infiltration.

PROCEDURE

Patient Assessment

1. Assess patient, catheter insertion site, and patient's extremities for signs of infiltration:
   - Inspect site around catheter tip and extremity for swelling, blanching, stretched and firm skin, or coolness.
   - Check for blood return or "flash" of blood. Blood return may be present although other signs of infiltration may be noted.
2. Question patient regarding pain, heat, and discomfort at access site.
3. Rate affected area using the **Infiltration Scale**. The scale provides a uniform standard for measuring the degree of infiltration.

GRADE	CLINICAL CRITERIA
0	No symptoms
1	Skin blanched Edema <1 inch in any direction Cool to touch With or without pain
2	Skin blanched Edema 1-6 inches in any direction Cool to touch With or without pain
3	Skin blanched, translucent Gross edema >6 inches in any direction Cool to touch Mild-moderate pain Possible "numbness" per patient
4	Skin blanched, translucent Skin tight, leaking Skin discolored, bruised, swollen Gross edema >6 inches in any direction Deep pitting tissue edema Circulatory impairment Moderate-severe pain Infiltration of any amount of blood products, irritant, or vesicant

Source: Infusion Nurses Society. Infusion Nursing Standards of Practice. *J Intravenous Nurs.*; 23(6S): S57.

Nursing Interventions

1. Provide patient with instructions on how to recognize signs and symptoms of infiltration.
2. Once infiltration is observed, discontinue infusion and remove catheter.
   - Apply pressure at removal site to prevent bleeding.
   - Depending on solution or medication infused, apply warm or cold compress to site to alleviate discomfort and help absorb infiltration by increasing circulation to affected area.
3. If leaking of the tissues occurs because of an extensive infiltration, apply a sterile dressing to the affected area. Remove dressing when drainage ceases.
4. Report infiltration rates of Grade 3 or 4 to physician.
5. Complete Unusual Occurrence Report as established by the organization.

Post Nursing Intervention

1. Document in patient's medical record.
2. When inserting new catheter, do not use affected (infiltrated) arm.
   - Use opposite extremity if possible.
   - Avoid areas of flexion.
   - Educate patient as to preventive measures as well as signs and symptoms of infiltration development.
3. Maintain statistical data on infiltration rates including degree, incidence, cause, and correction.

Infusion-Related Complications

Extravasation

CONSIDERATIONS FOR THE OLDER ADULT

Extravasation of vesicant parenteral solution or medication in the older adult can be particularly devastating. When a vesicant solution or medication extravasates, it can cause formation of blisters, with subsequent sloughing of tissues occurring from tissue necrosis.

The perception of cutaneous pain may decrease as a result of diminished receptors in aging skin. The older adult may have a change in peripheral sensations, causing decreased responses to stinging, heat or pain, or recognition of swelling at the venipuncture site resulting in more extensive injury.

Older adults tend not to report discomfort and pain as frequently as younger patients. Such patients can be accurately assessed when prompted more frequently. Special attention should be given to older adults who are unable to communicate verbally.

Older adults may feel they are expected to tolerate some level of pain. Expression of discomfort may be considered a weakness, he or she may fear being viewed as "difficult," or may fear that there is a serious reason for the pain such as disease progression and imminent death.

The body's capacity to heal can also be decreased due to age and disease processes. Infection is more likely to develop in damaged tissues and can lead to the need for surgery, loss of the extremity, and even death.

Extravasation can also contribute to medication error by delay of therapy administration and fluctuations in therapeutic medication levels secondary to delivery disruption.

POLICY

Nurses must be knowledgeable regarding the administration of vesicant solutions or medications, and the signs and symptoms of extravasation. Preventative measures and treatment at the onset of extravasation shall be initiated.

PROCEDURE

Patient Assessment

1. Assess patient, catheter insertion site, and patient's extremities for signs of extravasation.

2. Inspect site around catheter tip and extremity for swelling, blanching, bleb formation, stretched and firm skin, or coolness.

3. Question patient regarding pain, heat, stinging, burning, and discomfort at access site.

4. Consider type, concentration, and volume of vesicant infused into affected area. Antineoplastic agents, such as doxorubicin, can cause severe tissue necrosis when they extravasate. Other medications that can cause tissue necrosis are, but not limited to, dopamine, norepinephrine, high-dose potassium chloride, amphotericin B, and calcium and sodium bicarbonate in high concentrations, dilantin, 5FU.

5. Rate the affected area using the infiltration scale. Extravasation is always rated as Grade 4. See Infiltration Scale, p.75.

Nursing Interventions

Once extravasation is suspected:

1. Discontinue infusion immediately.
2. Notify physician and obtain specific orders to treat extravasation.
3. Administer specific antidote as ordered. Either keep catheter in place or remove catheter and inject antidote around the affected area as recommended by manufacturer.
4. If catheter must be removed:
   - Aspirate before removing catheter.
   - Apply pressure at removal site to prevent bleeding.
5. Apply ice to affected extremity for 24-48 hours. In the case of extravasation of vinca alkaloids, apply controlled heat to affected area, as directed by manufacturer.
6. Elevate affected extremity.
7. Encourage patient to resume normal activity with affected arm to prevent stiffness and discomfort.
8. When inserting new catheter, do not use affected arm. Avoid areas of flexion.

Post Nursing Intervention

1. Document the following in patient's medical record:
   - Date and time of extravasation
   - Catheter type and size used
   - Whether insertion site is new or preexisting
   - Drug administered, method of administration, and amount infused
   - Patient complaints or experience during the extravasation
   - Appearance of access site
   - Physician notification
   - Treatment and measures instituted
   - Outcome
2. With patient's consent, photograph affected area at the following intervals:
   - At time of injury
   - 24 hours after injury
   - 48 hours after injury
   - One week after injury
3. Complete Unusual Occurrence Report as established by the organization.
4. Maintain statistical data on extravasation rates, including degree, incidence, cause, and outcome.

Infusion-Related Complications

Allergic Reaction

> ### CONSIDERATIONS FOR THE OLDER ADULT
>
> An allergic reaction is a systemic or generalized hypersensitivity response to the administration of a solution, medication, or additive. Reactions may be immediate or delayed, mild to severe. If a reaction is severe enough, it can be life threatening. Common parenteral medications that can cause allergic reaction are antimicrobial agents, enzymes, and hormones. As an individual advances in years, the chance of developing various disease processes increases, leading to exposure to more drugs for treatment or intervention. The more drugs that the older adult is exposed to, the greater the risk for allergic reaction as well as adverse drug interaction occurrences.
>
> If an allergic reaction occurs, the causative agent shall be identified if possible, the infusion stopped, and the physician notified immediately. It is important when assessing the older adult to obtain a complete medication history and any documentation of past experiences with reactions or sensitivities, including over-the-counter medications, herbal remedies and culturally-biased preparations.

POLICY

The nurse shall be aware of signs and symptoms of allergic reactions and of patients who may be susceptible to allergic reactions.

PROCEDURE

Patient Assessment

1. Assess patient for signs and symptoms of allergic reaction.
   - Chills and fever with or without urticaria
   - Erythema
   - Itching
   - Shortness of breath with or without wheezing
   - Respiratory distress
   - Anaphylactic shock or cardiac arrest
2. Assess and monitor patient's vital signs.

Nursing Interventions

1. To prevent development of allergic reaction:
   - Obtain a thorough allergy and drug history; note any cross-sensitivity.
   - Place identification bracelet on patient noting allergy.
   - Flag patient's medical record to alert other healthcare professionals of patient's allergy.
   - Carefully perform patient identification during blood transfusion procedures.
2. If allergic reaction is suspected:
   - Stop infusion immediately.
   - Discontinue any medication suspected of causing reaction.
   - Maintain vascular access for emergency treatment. Have ready for immediate infusion 0.9% sodium chloride solution via new administration set.

- Notify physician immediately.
- Perform interventions and treatment as ordered.
- Administer antihistamines as ordered.
- Administer epinephrine or steroids as ordered.
- Monitor patient's vital signs.

Post-Nursing Intervention

1. Document the following in patient's medical record:
   - Observations and patient assessment
   - Physician notification
   - Interventions taken and outcome
   - Patient's condition and response to interventions
2. Complete an Unusual Occurrence Report as established by the organization.
3. Maintain statistical data on incidence of allergic reactions, cause, treatment, and outcome.

Infusion-Related Complications

Embolism: Air

CONSIDERATIONS FOR THE OLDER ADULT

Air embolism is a serious complication that occurs when air is inadvertently introduced into the catheter. The air may travel to the heart, causing pain, cardiac arrest or death. The older adult may not be able to articulate pain, palpitations, or other signs and symptoms associated with air embolism. Even if the patient is aware that something has changed, he or she may not be able to call for help due to preexisting conditions such as stroke, intubation or tracheotomy, or dementia and delirium.

If a central catheter becomes dislodged or disconnected, the older adult must be immediately assessed for signs of air embolism. Particular attention should be paid to the older adult at risk for inadvertent separation of the tubing from the VAD or removing the device entirely. Preparing the patient for removal of a CVAD is important but may not be completely understood by the older adult.

POLICY

Measures to prevent air embolism shall be routinely followed. Infusion equipment should use Leur-Lok™ attachment mechanisms to prevent inadvertant separation of the administration set. The nurse shall be knowledgeable concerning the prevention, signs and symptoms, and treatment of air embolism.

PROCEDURE

Patient Assessment

1. Assess patient for signs and symptoms of air embolism.
   - Chest pain
   - Complaint of shoulder or low back pain depending on the location of the embolus
   - Shortness of breath
   - Cyanosis
   - Hypotension
   - Weak, rapid pulse
   - Delirium
   - Syncope or loss of consciousness
   - Shock or cardiac arrest
2. Monitor vital signs.
3. Auscultate chest. A loud continuous churning sound may be heard over precordium.

Nursing Interventions

1. To prevent the formation of an air embolus:
   - Use air-eliminating filter on all infusion administration sets when and where appropriate during infusions.
   - Ensure that catheter and tubing are clamped during administration set change.
   - Use Leur-Lok™ connections on all add-ons and infusion equipment to prevent accidental separation.
   - Prime infusion sets, tubing and add-on devices with solution to be infused prior to attachment to VADs.

- Place patient in supine position; instruct and perform Valsalva maneuver during CVAD removal.
- Upon catheter removal, apply pressure to exit site; apply antiseptic ointment and occlusive dressing to catheter exit site.
- Change dressing and assess site every 24 hours until catheter exit site is epithelialized.

2. If air embolism is suspected:
   - Immediately place patient on the left side in Trendelenburg position; this will minimize migration of air embolus.
     - If air embolism results from open or leaking infusion system:
       - Clamp line close to access device to stop air intake.
       - Change solution container and tubing.
       - Support patient during resuscitation.
     - If air embolism results from disconnected or damaged CVAD:
       - Clamp catheter.
       - Repair catheter, if appropriate, according to manufacturer's recommendations. Otherwise, remove CVAD after inserting new catheter to support patient during resuscitation.
       - Notify physician immediately.
       - Continue to monitor vital signs and observe patient.
       - Perform interventions and treatments as ordered.
       - Administer oxygen as ordered.

Post Nursing Intervention

1. Document the following in patient's medical record:
   - Observations and patient assessment
   - Physician notification
   - Interventions taken and outcome
   - Patient's condition and response to interventions
2. Educate the patient on appropriate CVAD care and maintenance, recognition of signs of air embolism, and appropriate interventions to take in the event of an occurrence.
3. Complete Unusual Occurrence Report as established by the organization.
4. Maintain statistical data on incidence of air embolism, cause, treatment and outcome.

Infusion-Related Complications

Pulmonary Edema

CONSIDERATIONS FOR THE OLDER ADULT

Older adults often have compromised cardiac or renal systems which put them at particular risk. If the condition is not identified and immediately corrected, it can lead to congestive heart failure, shock, and cardiac arrest. The infusion of too much fluid, or at too rapid a rate, will often precipitate this complication. The older adult may not be able to articulate symptoms due to preexisting conditions such as stroke, intubation or tracheotomy, or dementia and delirium. Frequent monitoring of the older adult and all infusions is essential.

POLICY

Measures to prevent pulmonary edema shall be routinely followed. The nurse shall be knowledgeable concerning the signs, symptoms, and treatment of pulmonary edema.

PROCEDURE

Patient Assessment

1. Assess patient for early signs and symptoms of pulmonary edema.
   - Restlessness
   - Slow increase in pulse rate
   - Headache
   - Shortness of breath
   - Nonproductive cough
   - Skin flushing
   - Delirium
2. Assess patient for later signs and symptoms of pulmonary edema.
   - Hypertension
   - Severe dyspnea with "gurgly" or wet respirations
   - Coughing frothy fluids
   - Venous dilation as evidenced by engorged neck veins, pitting edema, moist rales
   - Puffy eyelids
3. Monitor patient's vital signs.

Nursing Interventions

1. To prevent development of pulmonary edema, carefully assess patient prior to receiving infusion therapy for:
   - History of problems associated with infusion therapy.
   - History of cardiac and respiratory problems.
   - Present fluid status relative to ability to tolerate fluid volume.
2. Monitor closely for tolerance of parenteral administration of solutions or medications.
   - Maintain fluid rates as ordered.
   - Use EID when administering solutions or medications that require accurate measurement.

3. If pulmonary edema is suspected:
   - Place patient on strict bed rest in high Fowler's position.
   - Slow infusion rate of solution or medication enough to maintain patency of VAD.
   - Notify physician immediately.
   - Monitor vital signs and fluid balance.
   - Perform interventions and treatments per physician's order.
   - Administer oxygen.
   - Administer pain medication.
   - Administer diuretics.
   - Administer vasodilators.
   - Perform phlebotomy.

Post Nursing Intervention

1. Document the following in patient's medical record:
   - Observations and patient assessment
   - Physician notification
   - Interventions taken and outcome
   - Patient's condition and response to treatment
2. Complete an Unusual Occurrence Report as established by the organization.
3. Maintain statistical data on incidence of pulmonary edema, cause, treatment and outcome.

Infusion-Related Complications

Speed Shock

CONSIDERATIONS FOR THE OLDER ADULT

Unlike pulmonary edema, speed shock may result from the infusion of smaller volumes of medication or solution. Speed shock usually results from the administration of a bolus medication or solution at a rapid rate. The older adult may not be able to articulate symptoms of dizziness, headache or other symptoms due to rapidity of onset. The rate of administration of any parenteral medication or solution must be carefully controlled and the older adult closely observed. Early symptoms can progress to tightness in the chest, hypotension, irregular pulse and anaphylactic shock.

POLICY

Measures to prevent speed shock shall be routinely followed. The nurse shall be knowledgeable concerning the signs, symptoms, and treatment of speed shock.

PROCEDURE

Patient Assessment

1. When administering medications, assess the patient for:
   - Dizziness
   - Facial flushing
   - Headache
   - Irregular heart rate
   - Sudden onset of symptoms associated with medication being administered
2. Continue to assess patient until infusion is completed.
3. Monitor patient's vital signs.

Nursing Interventions

1. To prevent the development of speed shock:
   - Monitor gravity-flow administration sets closely to ensure correct prescribed flow rate.
   - Use infusion control device when administering solutions or medications that require accurate measurement.
   - Follow recommended infusion rate of the medication.
2. If speed shock is suspected:
   - Stop the infusion immediately.
   - Maintain vascular access for emergency treatment.
   - Notify physician immediately.
   - Perform interventions and treatments per physician's order.
   - Monitor patient's vital signs.

Post Nursing Intervention

1. Document the following in patient's medical record:
   - Observations and patient assessment
   - Physician notification

- Interventions taken and outcome
- Patient's condition and response to intervention

2. Complete Unusual Occurrence Report as established by the organization.

3. Maintain statistical data on incidence of speed shock, cause, treatment, and outcome.

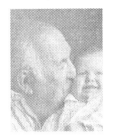

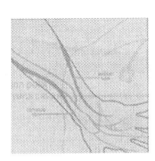

7.

Infusion Therapies

Hypodermoclysis

CONSIDERATIONS FOR THE OLDER ADULT

Hypodermoclysis therapy is the administration of isotonic infusates subcutaneously to correct short-term fluid and electrolyte disturbances. Isotonic fluid and electrolytes are administered subcutaneously upon a physician's or by a legally authorized prescriber's order. Hypodermoclysis may be indicated for short-term parenteral infusion therapy for the older adult who does not require emergent hydration therapy. Vascular routes for parenteral fluid delivery may be diminished or difficult to assess due to dehydration and previous insertion attempts. Other considerations should include:

- Fluid requirements less than 3000 mls/day
- No evidence of coagulation disorders
- Intact available skin sites

Hyaluronidase may be added to the infusate to aid in fluid absorption. The older adult should be tested for sensitivity to medication before initiating therapy via injection of subcutaneous dose. If hyaluronidase is not added to the infusate, absorption may be slowed and erythema at the clysis site may be observed.

POLICY

The nurse administering subcutaneous isotonic fluids and electrolytes shall be knowledgeable of the indications for use, appropriate rates of administration, monitoring parameters, side effects, stability of infusate, storage requirements, and potential complications.

PROCEDURE

Patient Assessment and Education

1. Verify patient's identity.
2. Obtain and review physician's order for type of fluid, amount, rate, route of administration, frequency and duration.
3. Plan patient's care.
4. Obtain patient's consent prior to therapy.
    - Obtain consent of legally authorized guardian if patient unable to give consent.
5. Educate patient (or legally authorized guardian) as to purpose and anticipated outcome of therapy, type of fluid, route of administration, signs and symptoms of complication recognition.
6. Assess patient.
    - Allergies
    - Obtain cardiac status.
    - Obtain baseline vital signs, weight and height.
    - Review laboratory data and assess for appropriateness of therapy.
    - Assess skin integrity at selected sites for subcutaneous administration.
7. Place patient in comfortable reclining position.

Prior to Beginning Procedure

1. Wash hands.
2. Assemble equipment.
3. Don gloves.
4. Use aseptic technique and observe Standard Precautions.

Insertion Site Selection

1. Assess sites for device placement.
   - Anterior and lateral aspects of thighs and hips
   - Upper abdominal wall
   - Subclavicular region
   - Dorsal aspect of upper arm
   - Subscapular region
2. Select insertion site with adequate subcutaneous tissue.
   - A fat fold of at least 1 inch or 2.5 cm. when forefinger and thumb are gently pinched together
3. Avoid areas of compromised integrity such as, but not limited to:
   - Edema
   - Pain
   - Excoriation
   - Infection
   - Bruise or hematoma
   - Scar tissue
4. Avoid areas located near
   - Breast tissue: fluid may drain into axillary lymph nodes.
   - Perineum: fluid may drain into scrotum or labia.
   - Within close proximity of umbilical area.
5. Avoid areas that may be prone to irritation from clothing and body motion.

Insertion Site Preparation

1. Wash insertion site with antiinfective soap and water if necessary.
2. Remove excess hair from intended insertion site with clippers or scissors (optional).
3. Disinfect insertion site with single-dose antiseptic solution. Recommended solutions include:
   - Chlorhexidine
   - 10% Povidone-iodine
   - Alcohol
   - 2% Tincture of iodine
4. Cleanse site using antiseptic solution.
   - Apply antiseptic solution according to manufacturer's recommendations for product use.
   - Work to anticipated dressing margin.
   - Allow antiseptic solution to air dry (do not blow or blot dry).

Device Selection and Insertion

1. Select access device with a 25-27 gauge ½-inch winged steel infusion set or 24 gauge ¾ -inch flexible catheter.

2. Attach administration set to infusate container and purge system.

3. Attach clysis infusion needle set to administration set and purge.
   • Inspect access device for defects.
   • Hang container above patient's head on IV pole.

4. Remove needle guard from set.

5. Lift skin into small mound.

6. Grasp infusion needle set and insert into prepared site.
   • 30°-45° for winged steel infusion set
   • 90° for infusion set with adhesive disk

7. Lay access device against skin (optional: secure with single piece sterile tape).

8. Observe for negative blood return. If blood return observed:
   • Remove device and select new insertion site.
   • Prepare new site.
   • Use new sterile clysis infusion set.

9. Apply TSM dressing over device shield.

10. Secure administration set tubing to skin to prevent accidental dislodgment.

11. Label dressing with device gauge and length, date and time, and initials of inserter.

Hypodermoclysis Administration

1. Only isotonic parenteral infusates are to be given subcutaneously.

2. Inspect fluid container for leaks, cracks, or particulate matter.

3. Initiate infusion at 30 ml/hour and monitor patient's response. If tolerance is noted, increase to prescribed rate after one hour.

4. Monitor patient's response and infusion site at regular intervals.

5. Observe for complication development.
   • Fluid overload
   • Erythema
   • Fluid leakage
   • Infection
   • Device dislodgment

6. Rotate site every 72 hours or sooner if complication(s) develop. Rotate site location at least 2-3 inches away from previous location to facilitate fluid absorption and decrease incidence of adverse effects.

7. If using gravity infusion system:
   • Open clamp.
   • Regulate flow of solution to infuse as ordered.

8. If using electronic infusion device (EID):
   • Prime tubing according to manufacturer's recommendations.
   • Follow manufacturer's recommendations for use of EID.

Post Insertion

1. Do not flush infusion device.
2. Discard used equipment and supplies.
3. Remove gloves.
4. Wash hands.
5. Document the following in the patient's permanent medical record:
   - Type of infusate administered
   - Volume and rate
   - Route of administration
   - Type of infusion controller
   - Date and time of administration
   - Skin integrity and location of clysis access site
   - Patient's education
   - Consent and response to procedure and therapy

Device Removal

1. Obtain and review physician's order for infusion discontinuance.
2. Wash hands.
3. Assemble equipment.
4. Don gloves.
5. Use aseptic technique and observe Standard Precautions.
6. Place patient in comfortable reclining position.
7. Clamp administration set and stop EID.
8. Remove transparent dressing and securement tapes.
9. Remove clysis administration set, activating safety mechanism; discard in sharps container.
10. Apply manual pressure with sterile gauze to prevent bleeding and fluid leakage.
11. Cover site with dry sterile dressing.
12. Discard expended equipment in appropriate receptacle(s).
13. Document the following in the patient's permanent medical record:
    - Type of infusate administered
    - Volume and rate
    - Route of administration
    - Type of infusion controller
    - Date and time of administration
    - Skin integrity and location of clysis access device
    - Patient's education
    - Consent and response to procedure and therapy

EQUIPMENT

General Supplies

- Antiseptic solutions
- Sterile 2x2 gauze pads
- Tape
- Gloves
- Disposal receptacle(s)
- Sharps container
- Receptacle for expended waste

Hypodermoclysis Therapy Supplies

- Infusate solution container
- Administration set
- Clysis access set
- Infusion controller (mechanical or electronic)

Parenteral Pain Management

CONSIDERATIONS FOR THE OLDER ADULT

Pain management medications and patient-controlled analgesia (PCA) are administered via continuous, intermittent, or combination infusions, upon the orders of a physician or legally authorized prescriber. Routes of parenteral pain medication administration include subcutaneous, intravascular, and intrathecal routes.

The perception of cutaneous pain in the older adult may decrease as a result of diminished receptors in aging skin in addition to neurological changes. However, perception of visceral pain may increase. Older adults with diagnoses of pain associated with malignancies may experience similar levels of pain intensity but require less analgesia.

Special attention should be given to older adults who are unable to communicate verbally. Older adults tend not to report discomfort and pain as frequently as younger patients. Older adults may feel they are expected to tolerate some level of pain. Expression of discomfort may be considered a weakness, he or she may fear being viewed as "difficult," or may fear that there is a serious reason for the pain such as disease progression and imminent death. Therefore, there is a tendency for nurses to undermedicate. Such patients can be accurately assessed when prompted more frequently.

Be sure the older adult is wearing glasses and hearing aids if appropriate as visual representations of pain measurement are more reliable than mental imaging.

Older adults will require more frequent assessments of pain and its management.

Side effects of pain medication administration may be more pronounced, such as constipation, sedation, or confusion. When assessing the older adult for pain and management thereof, the nurse should consider the possibility that the older adult may be delirious or anxious due to the existence of pain. The nurse should observe the patient for nonverbal indicators of pain such as grimacing, breathing irregularities, restlessness, crying, combativeness, and body posturing and rigidity.

POLICY

The nurse administering parenteral pain management shall be knowledgeable of the medications used for pain management, indications for use, appropriate dosage and diluents, administration, monitoring parameters, side effects, toxicities, incompatibilities, stability, storage requirements, potential complications, and both conventional and advanced methods of pain control.

PROCEDURE

Patient Assessment and Education

1. Verify patient's identity.
2. Obtain and review physician's order for medication, dosage, titration parameters, route of administration, frequency and duration.
3. Plan patient's care.
4. Obtain patient's consent prior to therapy initiation.
   • Obtain consent of legally authorized representative if patient is unable to give consent.
5. Educate patient on medication(s) and purpose and goal, route of administration, pump operation, side effects, monitoring parameters, and potential complications.

6. Assess patient.
   - Obtain baseline vital signs, weight and height.
   - Review laboratory results and assess for appropriateness of therapy.
   - Monitor patient for signs of respiratory depression, nausea and vomiting, pruritus, urinary retention, and hypertension.
   - Assess patient's response to pain medication using appropriate pain scale (See Appendix 3, Pain Intensity Scale).
   - Assess skin integrity at selected sites for subcutaneous administration.
7. Place patient in comfortable reclining position.

Insertion Site Selection and Device Placement

1. See Section 4, Site Selection and Device Placement (p.37).

Therapy Administration

1. Check medication label and inspect fluid container for leaks, cracks, or particulate matter.
2. Follow policy on Flushing (see Section 5, p.54) as appropriate.
3. Change administration set every 72 hours, immediately upon suspected contamination, or when system's integrity is compromised.
4. Connect administration set to access device.
5. Use electronic infusion device (EID).
   - Follow manufacturer's recommendation for use of EID.
   - Prime tubing according to manufacturer's recommendations.
   - Instruct patient or designated caregiver, as appropriate, on the use of PCA infusion device including operating instructions, expected outcomes, precautions, and potential side effects.
6. Document in the patient's medical record the type of fluid administered, medication administered, dosage, route of administration, rate of infusion, type of infusion controller, date and time of administration, and patient's response to medication and procedure.

EQUIPMENT

General Supplies

- Alcohol pads (see Intrathecal Pain Management Supplies, below)
- Tape
- Gloves
- Sharps container
- Receptacle for expended waste

Continuous Subcutaneous Pain Management Supplies

- Infusate solution or medication
- Administration set
- Infusion catheter
- Start kit
- Syringe: 5-cc size
- Preservative-free 0.9% sodium chloride, injection, 10-ml vial
- Electronic infusion device or PCA infusion device

Intravenous Pain Management Supplies

- Infusate solution or medication
- Administration set
- Infusion catheter
- Start kit
- Syringe(s): 3- or 5-cc sizes
- Preservative-free 0.9% sodium chloride, injection, 10-ml vial
- Electronic infusion device or PCA infusion device

Intrathecal Pain Management Supplies

No alcohol or acetone-based products are to be used; only preservative-free medications or solutions are to be infused.

- Infusate solution or medication
- Administration set with surfactant-free in-line filter
- Preservative-free 0.9% sodium chloride, injection, 10-ml vial
- Syringe(s): 3- or 5 cc sizes
- Sterile drapes: 2
- Sterile gloves: 2 pair
- Mask
- Povidone-iodine prep pads or swabs: 3
- Electronic infusion device or PCA infusion device

Pain Management Via Continuous Subcutaneous Infusion

CONSIDERATIONS FOR THE OLDER ADULT

Pain management medications and PCA are administered via continuously, intermittently, or a combination of both, upon the orders of a physician or legally authorized prescriber.

The perception of cutaneous pain may decrease as a result of diminished receptors in aging skin and neurological changes. However, perception of visceral pain may increase. Older patients with diagnoses of pain associated with malignancies may experience similar levels of pain intensity but require less analgesia.

Special attention should be given to older adults who are unable to communicate verbally. Older adults tend not to report discomfort and pain as frequently as younger patients. Older adults may feel they are expected to tolerate some level of pain. Expression of discomfort may be considered a weakness, he or she may fear being viewed as "difficult," or may fear that there is a serious reason for the pain such as disease progression and imminent death.Therefore, there is a tendency for nurses to undermedicate. Such patients can be accurately assessed when prompted more frequently.

Be sure the patient is wearing glasses and hearing aids if appropriate as visual representations of pain measurement are more reliable than mental imaging.

Older adults will require more frequent assessments of pain and its management.

Side effects of pain medication administration may be more pronounced, such as constipation, sedation, or confusion. When assessing the older adult for pain and management thereof, the nurse should consider the possibility that the older adult may be confused or anxious due to the existence of pain. The nurse should observe the patient for nonverbal indicators of pain such as grimacing, breathing irregularities, restlessness, crying, combativeness, and body posturing and rigidity.

POLICY

The nurse administering parenteral pain management shall be knowledgeable of the medications used for pain management, indications for use, appropriate dosage and diluents, administration, monitoring parameters, side effects, toxicities, incompatibilities, stability, storage requirements, potential complications, and both conventional and advanced methods of pain control.

PROCEDURE

Patient Assessment and Education

1. Verify patient's identity.
2. Obtain and review physician's order for medication, dosage, titration

    parameters, route of administration, frequency and duration.
3. Plan patient's care.
4. Obtain patient's consent prior to therapy initiation.
    • Obtain consent of legally authorized representative if patient is unable to give consent.
5. Educate patient (or legally authorized representative) on medication(s), route of administration, pump operation, side effects, monitoring parameters, and potential complications.

6. Assess patient.
   - Allergies
   - Obtain cardiac status
   - Obtain baseline vital signs, weight and height
   - Review laboratory results and assess for appropriateness of therapy.
   - Monitor patient for signs of respiratory depression, nausea and vomiting, pruritus, urinary retention, and hypertension.
   - Assess patient's response to pain medication using appropriate pain scale.
   - Assess skin integrity at selected sites for subcutaneous administration.
7. Place patient in comfortable reclining position.

Prior to Beginning Procedure

1. Wash hands.

2. Assemble equipment.

3. Don gloves.

4. Use aseptic technique and observe Standard Precautions.

Insertion Site Selection

1. Assess sites for device placement
   - Anterior and lateral aspects of thighs and hips
   - Upper abdominal wall
   - Subclavicular region
   - Dorsal aspect of upper arms
   - Subscapular region
2. Select insertion site with adequate subcutaneous tissue.
   - A fat fold of at least 1 inch or 2.5 cm. when forefinger and thumb are gently pinched together.
3. Avoid areas of compromised integrity such as, but not limited to:
   - Edema
   - Pain
   - Excoriation
   - Infection
   - Bruise or hematoma
   - Scar tissue
4. Avoid areas located near
   - Breast tissue: fluid may drain into axillary lymph nodes.
   - Perineum: fluid may drain into scrotum or labia.
   - Within close proximity of umbilical area.
5. Avoid areas that may be prone to irritation from clothing and body motion.

Insertion Site Preparation

1. Wash insertion site with antiinfective soap and water if necessary.

2. Remove excess hair from intended insertion site with clippers or scissors (optional).

3. Disinfect insertion site with single-dose antiseptic solution. Recommended solutions include:

- Chlorhexidine
- 10% Povidone-iodine
- Alcohol
- 2% Tincture of iodine

4. Cleanse site using antiseptic solution.
   - Apply antiseptic solution according to manufacturer's recommendations for product use.
   - Work to anticipated dressing margin.
   - Allow antiseptic solution to air dry (do not blow or blot dry).

Device Selection and Insertion

1. Select access device with a 25-27 gauge ½-inch winged steel infusion set or 24 gauge ¾-inch flexible catheter.
2. Attach administration set to infusate container and purge system.
3. Attach subcutaneous infusion needle set to administration set and purge.
4. Inspect access set for defects.
5. If using pole-mounted EID, hang medication container above patient's head on IV pole.
6. If using ambulatory EID, place infusion device on flat surface.
7. Remove needle guard from set.
8. Lift skin into small mound.
9. Grasp infusion needle set and insert into prepared site.
   - 30°-45° for winged steel infusion set
   - 90° for infusion set with adhesive disk
10. Lay wings or adhesive base flat against skin (optional: secure with sterile tape).
11. Observe for negative blood return. If blood return observed:
    - Remove infusion set and select new insertion site.
    - Prepare new site.
    - Use new sterile infusion set.
12. Apply TSM dressing over infusion set-skin junction.
13. Secure administration set to skin to prevent accidental dislodgment.
14. Label dressing with infusion set gauge and length, date and time, and initials of inserter.

Pain Management via Continuous Subcutaneous Infusion

1. Check medication label and inspect fluid container for leaks, cracks, or particulate matter.
   - Validate order, medication label, and EID settings with second nurse prior to initiation of therapy.
2. Initiate infusion at prescribed rate and monitor patient's initial response.
3. Monitor patient's response and infusion site at regular intervals.
4. Observe for complication development.
   - Infusion-related complications
   - Respiratory depression
   - Catheter-related complications
   - Erythema

- Fluid leakage
- Infection
- Device dislodgment

5. Change administration set every 72-96 hours, immediately upon suspected contamination, or when system's integrity is compromised.

6. Rotate access site location every 72-96 hours, at least 2-3 inches away from previous location to facilitate medication absorption and decrease incidence of adverse site effects.

7. Use EID.
   - Follow manufacturer's recommendation for use of EID.
   - Prime tubing according to manufacturer's recommendations.
   - Instruct patient on the use of PCA infusion device including operating instructions, expected outcomes, precautions, and potential side effects.

8. Use visual pain scale for pain measurement (see Appendix 3).

Post Insertion

1. Do not flush infusion device.

2. Discard used equipment and supplies in appropriate containers.

3. Remove gloves.

4. Wash hands.

5. Document the following in the patient's medical record:
   - Type of fluid administered
   - Medication administered
   - Dosage
   - Route of administration
   - Rate of infusion
   - Type of infusion controller
   - Date and time of administration
   - Gauge and length of access device
   - Location of access device and number of insertion attempts
   - Patient's response to medication and procedure

Device Removal

1. Obtain and review physician's order for infusion discontinuance.

2. Wash hands.

3. Assemble equipment.

4. Don gloves.

5. Use aseptic technique and observe Standard Precautions.

6. Place patient in comfortable reclining position.

7. Clamp administration set and stop EID.

8. Remove transparent dressing and securement tapes.

9. Remove subcutaneous infusion set and engage protective mechanism.

10. Apply manual pressure with sterile gauze to prevent bleeding and fluid leakage.

11. Cover site with dry sterile dressing.
12. Discard expended equipment in appropriate receptacle(s).
13. Document in the patient's permanent medical record
    • Medication administered
    • Concentration, volume and rate
    • Route of administration
    • Type of infusion controller
    • Date and time of administration
    • Skin integrity
    • Number of insertion attempts and location of subcutaneous infusion set
    • Patient's education, consent and response to procedure and therapy

EQUIPMENT
General Supplies
    • Antiseptic solutions
    • Sterile 2x2 gauze pads
    • Tape
    • Gloves
    • Receptacle for expended waste
    • Sharps container

Continuous Subcutaneous Pain Management Supplies
    • Medication container
    • Administration set
    • Start kit
    • Syringe, 5-cc size
    • Preservative-free 0.9% sodium chloride, injection, 10-ml vial
    • Subcutaneous infusion set
    • Electronic infusion device or PCA infusion device

Blood Specimen Collection

CONSIDERATIONS FOR THE OLDER ADULT

Laboratory assays are necessary to ascertain disease progress and management strategies. Consideration should be given to careful and creative integration of parenteral medication and infusate administration schedules in order to minimize venipuncture procedures. Coordination of specimen collection with catheter insertion procedures will minimize vein trauma while preserving future venipuncture sites. Careful site selection of venipuncture sites for laboratory assay procedures will also preserve venous access while minimizing vein trauma. (See Appendix 2, Older Adult Infusion Patient: Selected Peripheral Infusion Sites.)

Decreases in tissue turgor, changes in nerve conduction contributing to hypersensitive or delayed response to pain, and delayed wound healing will contribute to changes in skin integrity, bruising and hematoma development, skin tearing and infectious processes. Changes in physiologic coagulation functions or as a result of medication protocols will impact bruising and hematoma potential. Older adults may not comprehend education processes necessary to maintain hemostasis post-sampling procedures.

POLICY

Blood specimen collection for blood sample assay determination, donor collection, or therapeutic indications may be drawn:

1. peripherally via venipuncture.
2. from peripheral VADs at the time of insertion.
3. from CVADs.

The nurse participating in blood collection shall be competent and knowledgeable in collection practices. Blood specimen collection from a peripheral vascular access device is performed only at the time of initial insertion of the device. Blood specimens may not be drawn from an infusion administration set or proximal to an existing infusion site. An indwelling peripheral or midline catheter is not routinely used for blood specimen collection.

PROCEDURE

Patient Assessment and Education

1. Verify patient's identity.
2. Obtain and review physician's order for blood specimen collection. Note: Obtain and review physician's order for blood specimen collection from a VAD.
3. Plan patient's care.
4. Obtain patient's consent prior to blood specimen collection.
5. Obtain consent of legally authorized guardian if patient unable to give consent.
6. Provide patient or legally authorized representative with educational material or information regarding the procedure.
7. Assess patient.
   • Allergies
   • Review laboratory data and assess for appropriateness of therapy.
8. Place patient in comfortable reclining or seated position.

Prior to Beginning Procedure

1. Wash hands.
2. Obtain appropriate blood collection tubes, patient identification labels, and venipuncture equipment.
3. Don gloves.
4. Use aseptic technique and observe Standard Precautions.

A. From Peripheral Venipuncture

1. Position patient with arm extended from body and in a dependent position.
2. Apply tourniquet.
3. Select vein.
   - Follow policy on Site Selection (Section 4)
   - Veins in the antecubital fossa are the best choice for blood specimen collection: basilic, median cubital, median antebrachial, cephalic veins.
4. Disinfect intended venipuncture site (see policy on Insertion Site Preparation, p.45).
5. Insert needle of blood collection equipment at 45° angle, hold in place, and advance specimen tube positioned in barrel holder.
6. Observe for backflow of blood into tube.
7. Obtain desired amount of blood:
   - Nurse should be knowledgeable as to the order of the draw.
   - If more than one tube of blood is needed, change tubes slowly and steadily, taking care not to move needle in cannulated vein and cause patient undue pain or discomfort, or bleeding from venipuncture.
8. Release tourniquet.
9. Remove last tube from barrel holder and set aside.
10. Remove needle from vein, applying manual pressure at site with gauze until hemostasis achieved.
11. Label tubes prior to leaving patient's bedside.

B. From Peripheral Vascular Access Device

1. Apply tourniquet.
2. Select vein.
   - Follow policy on Site Selection (p.38).
   - Select the appropriate vein for intended infusion therapy, as catheter will be left in place post-blood collection.
3. Disinfect venipuncture site (see policy on Insertion Site Preparation, p.45).
4. Insert catheter (see policy on Catheter Placement, p.47).
5. Attach needleless adapter of blood collection equipment to catheter adapter, hold in place, and advance specimen tube.
6. Observe for backflow of blood into tube.
7. Obtain desired amount of blood (Note: Obtain blood specimens prior to initiating therapy).
   - If more than one tube of blood is needed, change tubes slowly and steadily, taking care not to dislodge catheter and cause patient undue pain or discomfort.
8. Release tourniquet.

9. Remove last tube from barrel holder and set aside.

10. Stabilize access device, apply dressing.

11. Remove blood collection equipment from adapter.

12. Attach purged infusion administration set or capped extension set.

13. Secure connection junctions.

14. Initiate therapy.

15. Label tubes prior to leaving patient's bedside.

C. From CVAD

1. Discontinue administration of all infusates into the CVAD prior to obtaining blood samples.

2. Check patency of CVAD by flushing with 3-5 ml preservative-free 0.9% sodium chloride, injection.

3. When drawing from multilumen catheters, the distal lumen is the preferred lumen from which to obtain specimen (or the lumen recommended by the manufacturer).

4. Blood samples may be collected from CVAD by syringe method or vacutainer, as recommended by the manufacturer of the CVAD.

5. Blood specimens collected from certain CVADs may be adversely affected by catheter composition or material; check with CVAD manufacturer for recommendations on product use.

• Using the vacutainer method:

1. Clamp catheter.

2. Attach needleless connector to vacutainer barrel holder.

3. Place blood tube into vacutainer holder, do not engage.

4. Disinfect injection/access port with alcohol.

5. Remove connector cover and insert connector into injection/access port.

6. Unclamp catheter.

7. Advance blood tube inside vacutainer holder to activate retrograde blood flow.

8. Hold tube in place until blood flow ceases: this is considered the "discard."

9. Clamp catheter and remove blood tube from vacutainer holder, leaving holder connected to injection/access port.

10. Discard blood tube immediately into appropriate container.

11. Insert second blood tube, unclamp catheter, and obtain blood specimen(s) as ordered.

12. After all samples are collected, clamp catheter.

13. Remove vacutainer holder and needleless connector from injection/access port.

14. Flush catheter (see policy on Flushing, p.54) using 5-10 ml preservative-free 0.9% sodium chloride, injection.

15. Resume infusion by aseptically reattaching administration set and continuing therapy as prescribed.

16. Label tubes prior to leaving patient's bedside.

Optional:

17. Remove expended injection/access port or cap and discard; clean catheter adapter with alcohol.

18. Aseptically attach new purged sterile injection/access port to catheter adapter.

19. Flush catheter (see policy on Flushing, p.54) using 5-10 ml preservative-free 0.9% sodium chloride, injection, followed with heparin according to organizational policy and manufacturer's recommendations for product use.

• Using the syringe method:

1. Clamp catheter.

2. Attach needleless connector to empty syringe.

3. Disinfect injection/access port with alcohol.

4. Remove connector cover and insert connector into injection/access port.

5. Unclamp catheter.

6. Withdraw 1.5-2 times fill volume of CVAD of blood, reclamp catheter.

7. Remove and discard syringe immediately into appropriate container.

8. Aseptically attach second syringe to catheter hub, size(s) to be determined by amount of blood needed.

9. Unclamp catheter.

10. Withdraw blood into syringe. (Note: several syringes may be needed to obtain required amount of blood.)

11. Reclamp catheter and remove syringe.

12. Flush catheter (see policy on Flushing, p.54) using 5-10 ml preservative-free 0.9% sodium chloride, injection.

13. Resume infusion by aseptically reattaching administration set and continuing therapy as prescribed.

14. Transfer blood to collection tubes or vials and rotate vials using appropriate needles or needleless system. Label tubes prior to leaving patient's bedside.

Optional:

15. Remove expended injection/access port or cap and discard; clean catheter adapter with alcohol.

16. Aseptically attach new purged sterile injection/access port to catheter adapter.

17. Flush catheter (see policy on Flushing, p.54) using 5-10 ml preservative-free 0.9% sodium chloride, injection, followed with heparin according to organizational policy and manufacturer's recommendations for product use.

18. Transfer blood to collection tubes or vials and rotate vials using appropriate needles or needleless system. Label tubes prior to leaving patient's bedside.

D. From Implanted Port

Blood for specimen collection may be drawn from implanted vascular ports.

1. Clamp extension set and remove injection/access port.

2. Attach empty 10-cc syringe to hub of extension tubing and unclamp.

3. Aspirate 3-5 cc of blood into syringe.

4. Reclamp extension set.

5. Remove and discard syringe immediately into an appropriate container.

6. Attach an empty syringe to extension tubing hub and unclamp.

7. Aspirate blood into syringe. (Note: several syringes may be needed to obtain required amount of blood.)

8. Clamp extension tubing and remove syringe with blood.

9. Transfer blood to collection tubes or vials and rotate vials using appropriate needles or needleless system.

10. Attach prefilled injection cap attached to 10-ml syringe containing preservative-free 10 ml 0.9% sodium chloride.

11. Unclamp catheter.

12. Flush with saline.

13. Clamp extension tubing and remove syringe.

14. Attach heparin-filled syringe, if appropriate, and unclamp catheter.

15. Flush with 3-5 ml heparin (100 u/ml), as appropriate (see policy on Flushing, p.54).

E. Difficult Draw from CVAD:

If blood does not flow into the blood tube or syringe:

1. Have patient change position, cough, move arm above head, or hold a deep breath.

2. Attempt to flush catheter with preservative-free 0.9% sodium chloride, injection, and attempt to withdraw blood again.

3. Check expiration date and integrity of tube; replace blood tube with a new one.

4. If still unsuccessful, notify physician.

5. Draw the blood specimen peripherally.

Post Blood Drawing

1. Monitor patient's response.

2. Discard used supplies in appropriate receptacles.

3. Label blood samples with:
   • Patient's name
   • Patient's ID number
   • Date and time of specimen collection
   • Nurse's initials

4. Send samples to testing laboratory.
   • Place blood specimen in sealed container for transport.
   • Label container with "BIOHAZARD" label.
   • Certain specimens may need to be placed on ice during transport; check with laboratory for confirmation.

5. Remove gloves.

6. Wash hands.

7. Document in patient's medical record, including amount of blood used for sampling and patient response to procedure.

EQUIPMENT
General Supplies
- Gloves
- Gauze pads
- Tape
- Sharps container
- receptacle for expended waste

Blood Drawing
- Collection vials or tubes
- Vacutainer tube holder
- Needleless adapter(s)
- Flush solutions:
  - 10 ml preservative-free 0.9% sodium chloride, injection, 2 vials
  - 5 ml heparin (100 u/ml), 1 vial
- Injection Cap(s)
- Syringes:
  - 5 ml (4)
  - 10 ml (number appropriate for sampling)
- Tourniquet
- Labels for tubes
- Transport containers

Site Disinfection
- Antiseptic solutions:
  - Chlorhexidine
  - 10% povidone-iodine
  - Alcohol
  - 2% tincture of iodine

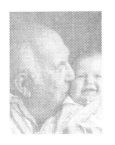

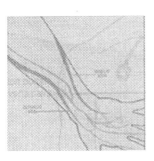

Appendix

Older Adult Infusion Patient Assessment: Systems Approach

Integumentary System	<ul><li>Loss of elasticity and thinning of surface tissues</li><li>Decreased subcutaneous fat</li><li>Increased skin surface dryness</li><li>Increased vascular fragility</li><li>Increased skin surface fragility</li><li>Decreased cell turnover</li><li>Decreased sweat glands</li><li>Slower wound healing</li></ul>
Immune System	<ul><li>Hyporesponsive to external stimuli</li><li>Decreased resistance to infections</li><li>Diminished ability to heal skin surface injuries</li><li>Deceptive signs of impending infection development</li></ul>
Musculoskeletal System	<ul><li>Decreased lean muscle mass leading to diminished capacity for mobility, strength and endurance</li><li>Erosion of cartilaginous surfaces leading to painful movement in all joint spaces</li><li>Decreased calcium absorption leading to osteoporosis</li></ul>
Digestive System	<ul><li>Decreased GI motility, mucosal atrophy, blood flow and increased gastric pH leading to impaired nutrient and vitamin absorption; early satiety affects fluid volume and food intake</li><li>Decreased hepatobiliary functions leading to decreased ability to metabolize medications and protein sources, decreased function in hematopoetic activities</li><li>Decreased salivation and decreased dentition leading to poor eating habits</li></ul>
Respiratory System	<ul><li>Impaired oxygen exchange contribute to delirium or restlessness</li><li>Increased risk of respiratory infections due to decreased elasticity of chest wall</li><li>Decreased muscle strength of diaphragm and intercostals muscles</li></ul>
Cardiovascular System	<ul><li>Slower response to fluid shifts including elimination of excess fluid</li><li>Venous and arterial insufficiencies</li><li>Decreased number of capillary beds</li><li>Decreased active functioning of venous valves resulting in diminished venous return</li><li>Decreased cardiac output and stroke volume</li><li>Increased rigidity of peripheral vasculature</li></ul>
Genitourinary System	<ul><li>Kidneys experience</li><li>diminished blood flow</li><li>decreased number of functioning nephrons resulting in decreased glomerular filtration rates and urine concentration, and</li><li>slowed creatinine clearance</li><li>Decreased bladder and capacitance sensation with increase in residual volume; relaxation of pelvic floor muscles causes increased risk of incontinence</li><li>Increased nocturnal urine elimination leads to disruption of sleeping patterns and sleep deprivation</li><li>Incontinence and physical immobility contribute to risk of urinary tract infections</li><li>Renal excretion of medication slowed causing reflex increase risk of untoward medication effects</li></ul>
Neurological System	<ul><li>Increased incidence of peripheral neuropathies, dementia, cerebral vascular accidents (CVAs)</li><li>Decreased number of neurons</li><li>Diminished neurotransmission activity results in changes in short-term memory</li><li>Decreased sensory functioning, slowed reflexes and increased visual and hearing deficits</li><li>Sensory and motor deficits contribute to increase in disability and potential loss of independence</li><li>Motor function deficits lead to coordination and balance impairments, resulting in orthostatic hypotension and increased risk of fall; slower reaction times during stressful activities</li><li>Pain may compromise capacity to cooperate effectively</li></ul>
Psychological and Environmental Assessment	<ul><li>Depression</li><li>Isolation as a result of physical impairment such as pain or sensory deficits, death of spouse/significant other or acting as primary caregiver to a disabled spouse/significant other</li><li>Delirium (acute change in mental status) as a result of foreign or unfamiliar surroundings from hospitalization or residence in care facility; potential for medication overdose when transported from home to healthcare facility due to compliance/financial issues</li><li>Communication difficulties due to disease, sensory deficits, cultural and language barriers</li></ul>

Older Adult Infusion Patient: Selected Peripheral Infusion Sites

Site	Veins	Advantage	Disadvantage
Hand	• Metacarpal • Dorsal venous arch • Inferior accessories of cephalic and basilic	• Easily accessible and visible • Accommodate most catheter gauge sizes • Distal location(s) • May not require support due to natural structures	• Uncomfortable secondary to autoimmune changes such as osteo- and rheumatoid arthritis • May impede activities of daily living (ADLs) such as self-care and handwashing, eating, use of ambulatory aids • Prone to skin tears and bruising
Forearm *dorsal and ventral surfaces	• Cephalic • Basilic • Median antebrachial	• Similar to "Hand" • Keeps hands free	• Difficult to observe and palpate in obese patient
Antecubital	• Cephalic • Basilic • Median	• Similar as for "Hand" • Keeps hands free • Larger veins visible and available for palpation • Preferred site for phlebotomy • Preferred site for Midline and PICC insertions	• Difficult to observe and palpate in obese patient • Antecubital region difficult to observe for complication development and management, ie, infiltration/extravasation, infection and bleeding • Limitations on activities such as ambulation and use of assistive devices, ADLs • Restrictions on phlebotomy • Limitations for potential future access for Midline or PICC insertion
Subcutaneous tissues (nonvascular)	• Subclavicular region (above breast tissue) • Abdomen • Upper thigh • Upper outer arm • Subscapula region	• Less discomfort (and agitation in cognitively impaired) • Fewer complications than with intravascular fluid administrations	• Infusion rate is slow • Local edema at site • Possible cellulitis at site

Adapted from: Hankins J., Lonsway RAW, Hedrick C., Perdue M. *Infusion Therapy in Clinical Practice*, 2nd edition. Philadelphia, PA: WB Saunders; 2001. P.580

Pain Intensity Guide

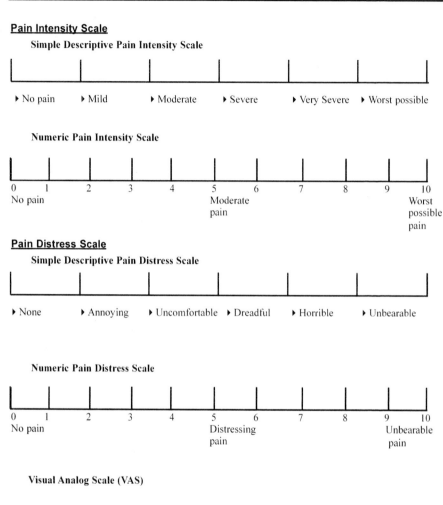

Pain Intensity Scale

Simple Descriptive Pain Intensity Scale

▸ No pain ▸ Mild ▸ Moderate ▸ Severe ▸ Very Severe ▸ Worst possible

Numeric Pain Intensity Scale

0 1 2 3 4 5 6 7 8 9 10
No pain   Moderate   Worst
     pain   possible
     pain

Pain Distress Scale

Simple Descriptive Pain Distress Scale

▸ None ▸ Annoying ▸ Uncomfortable ▸ Dreadful ▸ Horrible ▸ Unbearable

Numeric Pain Distress Scale

0 1 2 3 4 5 6 7 8 9 10
No pain   Distressing   Unbearable
     pain   pain

Visual Analog Scale (VAS)

No pain   Worst possible pain
or   *or*
no distress   Unbearable

Adapted from: AHCPR Acute Pain Management Guideline Panel. *Acute Pain Management: Operative or Medical Procedures and Trauma.* Clinical Practice Guideline. Rockville, MD: Agency for Health Care Policy and Research, Public Health Service, US Dept. of Health and Human Services. AHCPR Pub. No. 92-0032.

Resources and References

American Geriatrics Society: http://www.ags.org

Fetter, Marilyn S. Geriatric assessment and management protocols: issues for home infusion therapy providers. *J Infusion Nurs.* 2003;26(3):153-160.

Geriatric Depression Scale (GDS) available at:
http://www.stanford.edu/~yesavage/GDS.english.short.html

Hankins et al, eds. *Infusion Therapy in Clinical Practice,* 2nd edition. Philadelphia: WB Saunders; 2001.

Horgas, Ann L. Pain management in older adults. *J Infusion Nurs.* 2003;26(3):161-165.

Infusion Nurses Society. Clinical Competency Validation Program. 2003. INS, 220 Norwood Park South, Norwood, MA 02062.

Infusion Nurses Society. *Policies and Procedures for Infusion Nursing,* 2nd edition. 2002. INS, 220 Norwood Park South, Norwood, MA 02062.

Infusion Nurses Society. Infusion Nursing Standards of Practice. *J Intravenous Nurs,* 2000. 25(6S).

John A. Hartford Institute for Geriatric Nursing: http://www.hartfordign.org

Nurse Competency in Aging: http://www.geronurseonline.org.

Stechmiller, Joyce K. Early nutritional screening of older adults. *J Infusion Nurs.* 2003;26(3):170-7.

Whitehouse, M.J. Nursing assessment of the Older Adult. *J Intravenous Nurs.* 1992; 15(2S), suppl.: S14-S17.

Whitehouse, M.J. The physiology of aging. *J Intravenous Nurs.* 1992; 15(2S), suppl.: S7-S13.

Zwicker, C. DeAnne. The Older Adult at risk. *J Infusion Nurs.* 2003;26(3):137-143.